FAST FACTS FOR THE STUDENT NURSE

D0557456

About the Author

Susan Stabler-Haas, MSN, RN, CS, LMFT, is a registered nurse who has taught in diploma, associate, baccalaureate, RN-to-BSN, and second-degree nursing programs for more than 25 years. She has worked with students both in the classroom and at clinical sites. She currently teaches medical-surgical clinical nursing to senior baccalaureate students at West Chester University (West Chester, PA). She is the co-author of *Fast Facts for the Clinical Nursing Instructor* and has published articles on psychiatric nursing, relationship-based care, legal issues in nursing, and fundamentals of nursing. She has conducted research on the use of mindfulness-based stress reduction by nursing students.

Ms. Stabler-Haas is a diploma graduate of the Lankenau Hospital School of Nursing and holds both a baccalaureate and a master's degree in Nursing from Villanova University. Additionally, her education includes completion of a post-master's advanced practice program at the University of Pennsylvania. She has worked as a nurse and nurse-manager in the areas of critical care, medical-surgical, occupational health, and cardiac rehabilitation. Ms. Stabler-Haas is also a Clinical Nurse Specialist in adult psychiatric and mental health, and is a licensed marriage and family therapist.

FAST FACTS FOR THE STUDENT NURSE

Nursing Student Success in a Nutshell

Susan Stabler-Haas, MSN, RN, CS, LMFT

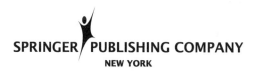

SPRINGER / PUBLISHING COMPANY

NEW YORK

610.7307
S775f

Springer Publishing Company, LLC
11 West 42nd Street
New York, NY 10036
www.springerpub.com

Acquisitions Editor: Allan Graubard
Composition: S4 Carlisle Publishing Services

ISBN: 978-0-8261-9324-7
E-book ISBN: 978-0-8261-9325-4

12 13 14/ 5 4 3 2 1

The author and the publisher of this Work have made every effort to use sources believed to be reliable to provide information that is accurate and compatible with the standards generally accepted at the time of publication. The author and publisher shall not be liable for any special, consequential, or exemplary damages resulting, in whole or in part, from the readers' use of, or reliance on, the information contained in this book. The publisher has no responsibility for the persistence or accuracy of URLs for external or third-party Internet Web sites referred to in this publication and does not guarantee that any content on such Web sites is, or will remain, accurate or appropriate.

Library of Congress Cataloging-in-Publication Data

Stabler-Haas, Susan.
  Fast facts for the student nurse: nursing student success in a nutshell/Susan Stabler-Haas.
    p. ; cm.
  ISBN 978-0-8261-9324-7—ISBN 0-8261-9324-2—ISBN 978-0-8261-9325-4 (e-book)
  I. Title.
    [DNLM: 1. Education, Nursing. 2. Students, Nursing. WY 18]
  610.7307—dc23

                                                                      2012006091

Printed in the United States of America by Hamilton Printing

10|13

Contents

Part III: Success at the Clinical Site

Part IV: Success at Home

Part V: Success Following Graduation

Foreword

When I heard Susan Stabler-Haas was writing a book to guide student nurses through the adventure that is nursing school, I was thrilled. Susan has an impressive array of clinical and nurse education experience, including a position as nurse manager in a medical intensive care unit, as a psychiatric clinical nurse specialist, and as an assistant professor of nursing and clinical instructor at West Chester University. As the "door is always open" professor with hands-on, diversified, and bedside experience, Susan Stabler-Haas is the perfect resource to assist students through the nursing school journey, knowledgeable on what it takes to succeed. As a recent graduate of nursing at West Chester University, I was fortunate enough to have benefited from Susan's guidance, understanding, and supportive mentoring as she offered her sound advice on studying, test taking, clinical success, and finding a job. Knowing how her guidance was a personal catalyst for success, the compilation of her expertise into a clear and concise guide will be an invaluable tool for future student nurses.

I vividly remember those times in nursing school, up to my ears in exams, term papers, and clinical reports, and feeling a loss of direction, blurred expectations, and the vague idea of "success" far away. I remember fingering through pages and pages of notes from lectures and feeling overwhelmed. How could there only be 50 questions on the next exam with this seemingly endless information? How can I study all of this?

I remember reading the project assignment for the dreaded term paper and pondering, what are the professors looking for? What is significant and relevant? Or the anxiety of starting clinicals, trying to finish the mandatory tasks but unsure of how to take advantage of the hands-on experience. I also remember the realization, as a college student, of how training for this job affected people's lives in a significant way and the necessary embrace of this new responsibility. I remember my feelings being shared by other students around me as these concerns proved to be universal in the transition to student nurse. Luckily, I had Susan as a member of my personal journey, assisting me through the challenge and guiding me through these unknown waters.

Nursing school is a unique and rewarding experience with new and distinct challenges. Navigating these challenges without guidance and attempting to "figure it out" alone as school progresses can hinder a student's potential. From lectures to clinical experiences, studying the dignified profession of nursing takes commitment, dedication, and a desire to succeed. Utilizing guidance in the form of this book can be highly beneficial for students who aspire to be professional nurses and bridges the desire with success in the classroom and clinical field. There are limited comprehensive resources available for nursing students such as this book, which includes chapters on classroom and clinical tips, working, and finding a job.

Take advantage of this book. Read it, highlight it, underline it, and study it. By using the information provided, you can feel in control of your nursing school experience, evolving into that capable nursing student of whom you can be proud. Nursing school is not easy, but being prepared and navigating through the numerous facets of curriculum and expectations with insider tips from a knowledgeable nursing school professor will surely set you up for success.

Laura Giambattista, RN, BSN
Clinical Nurse II
University of California
San Diego Medical Center

Preface

It had been a day like any other in the life of a seventh grader. My night had been unremarkable as well. But as I settled into bed and pulled the covers up around me, an event would occur that would one day help shape my professional life. While waiting for sleep to come, I heard the lonely and faraway cry of an ambulance. I listened as it crept closer and closer – slowly at first but then flying past my window like a Halloween ghost. I listened as its intense and mournful wail was gradually overcome by the returning stillness of the night. The ambulance had not stopped at my house, but it had managed to plant a seed in the imagination of a 12-year-old girl as it hurried by. To myself, I said, "I wonder what it would be like to be a nurse and help those who are sick."

It is curious how the most innocuous of events or the most casual of encounters can put us on a career path with no warning to ourselves and little notice by others. What made you interested in nursing as a career? Perhaps a family member or adult you admire worked as a nurse. Maybe you or someone close to you was a hospital patient, and you were intrigued by the nurses who constantly moved in and out of the room. You may have even read stories about how these wonderful and at times heroic individuals effectively combine the science of health care with the art of healing in the interest of making their patients well again. As noted in Chapter 8, "*Today's nurse is in constant motion, shuttling back and forth between the technical aspects of nursing practice and the human aspects of nursing care. There are few other professions that require their practitioners to be so adept in so many different ways. As a nurse, you can treat, educate, console, bathe, and medicate a patient all within the same day."*

Now poised to begin your life's work, you may have recently entered nursing school or are considering the possibility of becoming a nursing student. This book has been written especially for you. Its purpose is to acquaint you with the demands and rewards of both an education and a career as a nurse. Think of this book as a map of sorts that is intended to prepare you for the realities you will encounter as you embark upon your career journey. By knowing what to expect, you will be in a better position to navigate the sometimes turbulent and sometimes tranquil seas that now separate you from a nursing license.

You should first understand the perspective from which this book has been created. It is not the product of statistical research. Rather, it is a personal blend of informed observation, practical advice, and helpful hints from my experience as a staff medical-surgical nurse, a rehab nurse, an industrial nurse, a nurse manager in a critical care unit of a major urban hospital, a nurse psychotherapist, a nursing instructor in associate, diploma, and second-degree programs, a university assistant professor – and, yes, my own vivid recollections of having once been a student nurse myself. This book also represents experiences drawn from more than a thousand nursing students whom I have taught over the years. Many examples in this book are their stories, and the section at the end of each part entitled "In Student Nurses' Own Words . . ." are the real words of my former students.

I hope that this book will be your companion as you move through your nursing education program and eventually into your own nursing role. I also hope that it helps you to sustain your own mental and physical health as you progress toward your professional goal.

Finally, it is my fondest hope that you will find nursing to be both professionally and personally fulfilling, just like the girl who heard the ambulance race by her window so many years ago.

Acknowledgments

I would like to thank the many students whom I have had the privilege of teaching throughout my career. It is their diligence and commitment to succeed in the nursing profession that have provided the inspiration for this book. In particular, I would like to recognize two former students—Laura Giambattista, RN, BSN (who wrote the Foreword) and Kelly Dulik, RN (who provided added insight regarding the nursing student perspective).

In addition, I must pay homage to my own mentors who have helped to shape my future in the nursing profession, especially Lee Camera, Lynn Garonski, Sally Russo, and Susan Slaninka.

Of course, no acknowledgment is complete without recognizing the invaluable support of my family and friends, whose encouragement has sustained me in my quest for success as a nurse, teacher, and author. Last, thank you to my husband Joe, whose kind wisdom and suggestions added immeasurable value to this book.

PART

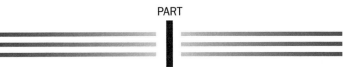

Your New Life as a Student Nurse

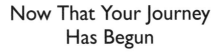

Now That Your Journey Has Begun

INTRODUCTION

A career in nursing is a journey that begins with information gathering and planning on the part of the student nurse.

In this chapter, you will learn:

1. That a career in nursing requires careful preparation.
2. About the public's perception of the nursing profession.
3. About the "typical" nursing student.

A CAREER IN NURSING REQUIRES CAREFUL PREPARATION

Think back to your last vacation. Was it fun? Did you relax? Was it everything that you hoped it would be? If so, chances are that your vacation's success was the result of careful planning—where to stay, what to pack, and, most important, how to get there.

In a larger sense, the mechanics of planning a career are similar to those involved in planning a vacation. Like those glossy brochures touting the many treasures and pleasures to be found from Las Vegas to London and from Madrid to Macao, a wide array of careers has beckoned to you. After carefully considering those options, you have decided that nursing is the profession that best reflects your personal values and ambitions.

THE PUBLIC'S PERCEPTION OF THE NURSING PROFESSION

Congratulations on making a great career choice! A 2010 Gallup poll has again found nursing to be the profession most trusted by the general public. Since becoming a part of this survey in 1999, nursing has been rated the most trusted profession every year with the exception of 2001, when firefighters took the top spot. The public's trust in nurses is well placed. In addition to being caregivers, nurses are often advocates for their patients, doing what they can to help them successfully navigate the health care system. It is a trust that can be traced back to the battlefield and the contributions of nursing icons such as Florence Nightingale and Clara Barton. Chances are, however, that you were drawn to the profession by an individual who is not famous—one whose skill and dedication kindled a passion within you strong enough to illuminate your ultimate career path.

THE TYPICAL NURSING STUDENT

The typical nursing student is no longer typical. Once she was almost exclusively a young white female, but that is changing. In 1990, minority enrollment in basic registered nursing programs was 16%; this nearly doubled to 29% by 2008–2009. Similarly, male participation has doubled as well, from a level of 6% in 1988 to about 12% today. The next threshold to be crossed is age. The advent of second-degree programs to accommodate career changers interested in nursing will no doubt begin to raise the average age of the nursing student as well.

FAST FACTS in a NUTSHELL

- A career in nursing requires careful preparation.
- Nursing is continually rated as society's most re-spected profession.
- The profile of the typical nursing student is evolving to become more inclusive of males, minorities, and older program participants.

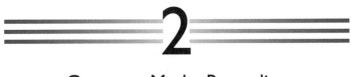

2

Common Myths Regarding Nursing

INTRODUCTION

As you imagine yourself as a nurse, be sure that your expectations separate fact from fiction.

In this chapter, you will learn:

1. Ten perceptions regarding the nursing profession.
2. Truth versus myth.
3. The importance of having a real-world perspective.

Now, having stepped onto a career path with your formal enrollment in a school of nursing, your focus should be on how to reach your destination safely. Over the course of your nursing education, there will be opportunities to be grasped and pitfalls to be avoided. Anticipating and planning for them will give you a distinct advantage as you gradually move closer to your goal. Therein lies the purpose of this book: to let you know what you can expect on your journey to become a nurse.

Nurses are a vital part of today's health care system, and tomorrow's as well. The nursing role is multidimensional. It requires an in-depth knowledge of physiology and pharmacology along with the insight and empathy to effectively interact with patients who are afflicted physically, mentally, and emotionally. Let's see what your perceptions are about becoming a nurse, and then determine if they are true.

TEN PERCEPTIONS REGARDING THE NURSING PROFESSION

TRUE OR FALSE ? ? ? ?

_____ I will make a lucrative salary as a nurse.

_____ It is easy to find a job as a nurse.

_____ Patients will always be grateful and positive to me.

_____ If I do well in my nursing class work, I will do well in my clinical rotation.

_____ If I am organized, I can always plan and predict my workday as a nurse.

_____ I like people, so I will like working with all of my patients.

_____ I will have nursing aides who will handle all of the "messy" parts of nursing.

_____ I would prefer to be a physician but becoming a nurse is much easier.

_____ I am going to become a nurse anesthetist or a nurse midwife following nursing school.

_____ I can keep my full-time job because my classes are on weekends and evenings.

TRUTH VERSUS MYTH

If you answered "false" to each of these questions, then give yourself an "A" grade. Although these perceptions are commonly held, they are not based in fact. Let's examine each of these myths individually.

MYTH 1   I Will Make a Lucrative Salary as a Nurse

While the initial salary may seem lucrative for a new graduate, the salary range itself tends to be relatively flat as one gains experience. Keep in mind that that an average salary includes holidays, weekends, and off shift (nights and evenings). After years of steadily increasing, beginning salaries for staff nurses have leveled off.

While the personal rewards of nursing can be great, this is truly a profession that one should not enter into "for the money" only.

MYTH 2   It Is Easy to Find a Job as a Nurse

Ten to fifteen years ago, new nurses could count on signing bonuses as health care facilities openly competed for their services. But times change. Recently, a health care system just outside of Philadelphia had 700 applications for 70 new nursing positions. In the last several years, the nursing job market has tightened considerably. Why? Like other professions, nursing is not immune to economic pressures. Many nurses who had planned to retire have had to change plans in the face of dwindling retirement funds, unemployed spouses, and adult children who are financially unable to subsist on their own. Additionally, there are now more nursing students than ever before. A study by the Robert Wood Johnson Foundation found that in 2010, enrollment in traditional nursing baccalaureate programs had increased by 5.7% over the prior year—the tenth consecutive year that an increase had been identified!

Like other professions, the job market for nursing will wax and wane over time. Despite high grade point averages and even personal connections, you will need careful planning and diligent effort to procure your first professional nursing position.

MYTH 3   Patients Will Always Be Grateful and Positive to Me

Most patients will be grateful and positive but don't depend on receiving their accolades every day! You may be caring for patients at one of the worst times in their lives. They are often experiencing pain or some other form of discomfort. They may also be very anxious, particularly if they believe (correctly or incorrectly) that their malady is life-threatening. Families that are under stress usually bring this stress with them to the critical care units, the med-surg floors, and the maternity units. If some family dysfunction already exists, it will often be manifested at the care site. Remember that there will be times that you are seeing patients and their families at their very WORST.

Fortunately, these occasions are the exceptions. Most patients will be happy to have you care for them. Most patients will be very grateful for the kind and caring service that you bring to them during their most difficult life events. But people are human and sometimes prone to be less than cordial. With that in mind, expect to have occasional unpleasant experiences with the people that you care for.

MYTH 4   If I Do Well in My Nursing Class Work, I Will Do Well in My Clinical Rotation

Some students who receive As on nursing exams may not recognize the gravity of a "real world" situation, resulting in a delay in procuring assistance for the patient.

Classroom exams tap the brain's memory and learning skills. Many nursing students have the innate ability to be good test takers—they have the cognitive skills to easily digest classroom content and commit it to memory. Clinical skills, however, are very different. While they obviously depend on your class work as a foundation, clinical skills also require superior analytical aptitude, psychomotor abilities, and emotional intelligence.

These different skills are needed at the clinical site. In the clinical education setting, students need to apply classroom knowledge to real-world situations. The hypothetical congestive heart failure patient you studied in the classroom is now right in front of you and not able to breathe. Are you able to assess and implement life-saving strategies immediately, which include recognizing the seriousness of the situation and informing your instructor and the primary nurse?

Clinical competence also requires psychomotor skills of assessment, bathing, performing complex nursing procedures, supervising intravenous therapies, and so on. Book knowledge will translate into performance only with experience, and the duration of that learning curve will vary from one individual to another as they are exposed to different patient situations.

Last, there is the aspect of emotional intelligence, which can be loosely described as the ability of an individual to accurately discern the feelings of another in the course of an encounter. The concept was popularized by Daniel Goleman (2009) in his book *Emotional Intelligence*. As a nurse, you will find that much of what is wrong or worrying a patient will be unspoken. Patients often do not know what to say to health care professionals and may actually be fearful to tell them about a certain pain. Will they keep me in the hospital if I tell them I felt faint when I first got up this morning? It takes emotional intelligence to recognize and seize upon those subtle cues offered by a patient as to what is really wrong, and to know what to say and how to say it in response.

So, despite its obvious importance, classroom success does not always guarantee clinical success.

MYTH 5   If I Am Organized, I Can Always Plan and Predict My Workday as a Nurse

An instructor found a senior nursing student in tears after one of her patient's medications was not available from the hospital pharmacy. The student said, "I work fine until something goes wrong." Nurses need to be flexible. Every day, about ten times a day in your life as a nurse, something will go wrong. It is imperative to have a plan, to be organized, to keep multiple patients' needs and priorities in your mind, and to keep track of them all. And yet, no matter how organized or prepared you may think you are, something is bound to happen that will require you to readjust your plans. While it is important to be organized, it is also important to be adaptable as you encounter the unplanned occurrence.

MYTH 6   I Like People, So I Will Like Working With All of My Patients

It is a good beginning to like people. But even the most compassionate of nurses will at times struggle to like the person whom he or she is required to care for. Are you irritated by chronic complainers? Are you put off by those who do little or nothing to promote their own health? Does the person in the hospital bed remind you of that neighbor or relative that you can't stand to be around? Remember that you are only human, and we humans all have our own individual triggers. Also remember that while the human in you may not like a particular patient, the professional in you must never let that show. You must still deliver the best care possible at all times.

MYTH 7   I Will Have Nursing Aides Who Will Handle All of the "Messy" Parts of Nursing

Nursing aides are unlicensed personnel who assist other team members in providing patient care to all clients. At best, some facilities will have one aide per one or two nurses. At the other end of the spectrum, other facilities will employ one aide for a whole floor of 30 patients. Staffing patterns can change by facility and from day to day in the same facility. Don't continue in the pursuit of a nursing license if you think that designation will allow you to avoid "getting your hands dirty." They will get dirty. Expectations in this regard are discussed later in the book.

MYTH 8   I Would Prefer to Be a Physician but Becoming a Nurse Is Much Easier

Please do not enter nursing school as a substitute for medical school. First, the professions and their concomitant responsibilities are very different. Physicians are responsible for determining a medical diagnosis and devising a medical treatment plan. Nurses are responsible for the total care—the mind, body, and spirit—of their patients. It often is the nurse who is the spokesperson for the client/patient to a physician.

Second, nursing school is challenging. Nursing education results in a thorough understanding of the body's functions and pathologies, and can prove very difficult. It would be a mistake to underestimate the degree of effort that nursing school will entail.

MYTH 9   I Am Going to Become a Nurse Anesthetist or a Nurse Midwife Immediately Following Nursing School

It is always fun to imagine your career trajectory but remember to investigate each stop you plan to make along the way! To apply to nurse anesthesia school, you need at least a year or two of critical care nursing, which is emergency department or intensive care unit nursing. Entrance into nurse anesthesia school is very competitive, so you need good references and solid experience. Similarly, nurse midwives are first required to have labor and delivery room experience and medical surgical experience as well. Give yourself some time to make a prudent decision as to how you will spend your nursing career. Your outlook will evolve as you continue in your nursing program. The person you are as you enter may not be the same person that exits. You may be surprised how your initial plans change once you complete nursing school. Keep an open mind and allow yourself to look at every opportunity.

MYTH 10   I Can Keep My Full-Time Job Since My Classes Are on Weekends and Evenings

The need to pay your bills is an inescapable reality. At the same time, have an accurate idea of the toll that working can take on your ability to successfully navigate a nursing education program. In nursing, your study transcends the simple need to pass the next exam. In fact, the knowledge you need to acquire is vital to the care you will one day render to your patients. At the risk of sounding dramatic, it is a simple truth that your patients' lives will be in your hands. So do not make the mistake of working too many hours in the course of your nursing education. Your student nurse role will demand a great deal of your energy. If you need to work full-time, you should reevaluate your decision to begin a nursing program now.

THE IMPORTANCE OF HAVING
A REAL-WORLD PERSPECTIVE

This is an important juncture in your life. Choosing a career path entails a significant investment of time and money. As a prospective nurse, begin with a clear and accurate understanding of what your role will be. Don't rely on the caricatures of the entertainment world to define what a nurse is. Talk to those already in the field and discover the demands and rewards of the real world on your own.

FAST FACTS in a NUTSHELL

- There are many misconceptions regarding the profession.
- It is important to uncover the reality beneath the myth.
- A student nurse with a real-world perspective will be better equipped to tackle the demands of the nursing profession.

3

Facing the Challenge of Your Chosen Major

INTRODUCTION

The rigor of the nursing major should be understood and appreciated by the nursing student.

In this chapter, you will learn:

1. The types of courses that a nursing education requires.
2. How a nursing major differs from other majors.
3. If you are equipped to be a nurse.

As the wedding guests were streaming to the dance floor, Bill's mother strained to be heard over the booming beat of the band. "I am worried about Bill. He started as a business major. He made it only as far as his sophomore year before he realized he would not pass. So, he decided to switch his major to nursing because he figured that would not be as difficult.

Guess what? He said nursing was even more difficult! Can you believe that? I don't know what he will do now."

THE TYPES OF COURSES THAT A NURSING EDUCATION REQUIRES

Pity poor Bill. If only he had made the effort to learn what it took to graduate with a nursing degree, he may have made a different choice in selecting an alternate major. He would have discovered that the nursing major demands proficiency in a number of technical courses. Below is a list of courses commonly found in the nursing curriculum, with a brief description of each:

Anatomy and physiology	Study of the human skeleton, muscles, and organs
Biology	Study of all basic life, including cellular structures and metabolism
Chemistry	Study of the theory and principles governing atomic structure, bonding, and reactions
Microbiology	Microscopic study of bacteria, fungi, viruses, etc., and their relationship to disease
Pathophysiology	The study of disease conditions in a physiological context
Pharmacology	Study of medications, their properties, their actions, and the nursing responsibilities associated with their delivery
Statistics	Study of mathematically based probability theory
Research	The application of statistics and relevant studies to support the efficacy of evidence-based nursing practice

HOW NURSING DIFFERS FROM OTHER MAJORS

Sure, every academic discipline has its own specialized courses. There is, however, an added dimension faced by the nursing student. In the course of your education, you will be asked to put what you have learned into practice by working in a hospital or other clinical setting under the direction of a nursing instructor. But, you may say, don't many other majors have the same requirement? After all, student teachers provide instruction in the classroom as part of their career preparation. Additionally, cooperative education in-office experiences are relatively common for business and technical students. So what's different about nursing?

What is different is the fact that your experience will require you to interact with strangers in a very personal way as you monitor their disease conditions and bodily functions. Inherent in this interaction is the degree of harm that a nursing student can potentially cause if he or she does not exercise appropriate caution. Simply put, without proper oversight on the part of the instructor and preparation on the part of the student, the student nurse can cause serious harm to a patient. That reason alone should provide you with any needed motivation to take your in-class instruction and your out-of-class studying seriously.

Responsible nursing programs understand the gravity of this responsibility and will not put you in a position to fail. Like any other student, you are human and mistakes are common to the practitioner of any new endeavor, including nursing. As a result, precautions are taken by your program and the clinical site wherever possible to avoid the occurrence of errors. But all of their risk avoidance measures can fall short if you do not do your part. Within the clinical setting, you have the duty to carefully put into practice what you do know, and to defer to your instructor or co-assigned staff nurse when you encounter a situation where your knowledge is lacking.

AM I EQUIPPED TO BE A NURSE?

Choosing nursing as your field is a life decision. As with any life decision, the voice of trepidation will occasionally whisper to you. For nursing students, that voice will sometimes ask, "Is this the right profession for me? Will I enjoy it? Will I be able to handle it?" Don't close your mind to that voice. It is an internal compass that you were born with to ensure that your life decisions keep you on a path that will lead to happiness.

Allow that voice time to speak to you. In truth, some will correctly conclude that nursing is not their field after all. Most students, however, will learn to enjoy and love the field more as they move deeper into their studies. Often this begins when students finally complete their prerequisite sciences and enter into their nursing courses. The feeling of commitment is then magnified in the clinical rotations involving nursing interaction with fellow human beings. This initial immersion into the world of nursing many times will kindle the personal revelation to students that all of their preparatory study has been worth it.

Too bad that our friend Bill did not pose this question to himself at the outset of his nursing studies. An honest self-appraisal on his part would have saved him some time and money, and opened his spot to someone who was better positioned to succeed. So what about you? Are you willing to undertake the educational effort associated with understanding the body's systems and attendant diseases? Are you willing to accept the responsibility of providing medical care to another human being? If you answered "yes" to these two questions, then read on. You are already on your way to becoming a good nurse.

═══════════════════════════════*FAST FACTS in a NUTSHELL*

- Nursing education has a strong technical component.
- Educational experiences outside the classroom require careful preparation on your part.
- Your success in the nursing program depends on your personal commitment.

In Student Nurses' Own Words . . .

"I was a bit overwhelmed in the beginning, but now I like nursing a lot more."

"I'm still really excited to be a nurse. I transferred into the program and it was difficult, but I'm so happy I stuck with it."

"I am excited to use the skills I have learned, but also a little nervous."

"I feel even more sure that nursing is the profession for me."

"It's definitely going to be difficult, but I like it and am going to stick with it."

"It is scary but also exciting."

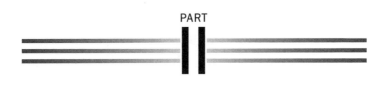

Success in the Classroom

4

Optimizing the Value of Classroom Time

INTRODUCTION

The conceptual knowledge you will need as a nurse is acquired in the classroom. As a result, deriving the maximum value from your classroom experience is essential to your professional success. Success in the classroom is not accidental. Rather, it is the result of preparation and organization on your part.

In this chapter, you will learn:

1. Helpful steps to take before class begins.
2. The importance of classroom logistics.
3. How to stay focused during class.

HELPFUL STEPS TO TAKE BEFORE CLASS BEGINS

In the course of her legendary career, singer Celine Dion once completed a four-year run of over 700 sold-out performances in Las Vegas. And yet, despite her magnificent talent, Ms. Dion held a rehearsal before every single show. She would not dare risk performing at less than her very best by relying on talent alone. Her top performance always required careful preparation.

Your life, of course, is not as glamorous, but the need for preparation is no different. For example, according to the course syllabus provided at the beginning of the semester, you will be introduced to the intricacies of the renal system tomorrow at 8:00 a.m. In the confines of a single hour, you will receive a significant amount of technical information that will wash over you like an ocean wave. How much of it will you absorb? That answer can vary in concert with the amount of preparation you are willing to invest prior to the lecture.

Preclass reading of the material to be covered for the next day's lecture is a MUST! Maybe you were able to pass prior exams in high school or your first college major by just listening in the classroom or studying the PowerPoint slides the night before the test. That was then—this is now. It won't work well for you or your patients if that is your plan for success as a student nurse. Here is your new strategy in preparing for class:

- Read the section of your textbook that pertains to the upcoming class.
- Create an outline from your reading in a notebook or laptop that you bring to class.
- Make a list of questions for anything that you have difficulty understanding.
- If the lecture does not eliminate your confusion, raise your hand and ask for clarification.

It is also a good idea to consult the syllabus for the objectives of the class. The listed objectives are the building blocks of the lecturer's notes and often provide the scaffolding for their content.

Realistically, you will not always have time to tackle all required readings for nursing courses from beginning to end.

You can, however, skim the material in advance to familiarize yourself with the terms you will encounter. Skimming is a skill that improves with practice. Compare the stated objectives of the upcoming lecture with the required reading assignment from the textbook or online source for this lecture. Focus on the chapter titles and subtitles that pertain directly to the objectives mentioned in the lecture topic's outline. Try to avoid the tempting shortcut of relying on printed slides that will accompany the lecture. Rarely are they sufficient in preparing you to grasp both the extent and the complexity of health conditions with which you must become familiar.

Often, just having a sense of the lecture topic to be covered is a step in the right direction. If too little information is available before the lecture day, email the instructor asking for guidelines for preparation. Most instructors will be pleased that you are taking the lecture time so seriously and will be happy to help you.

Finally, don't forget to get a good night's sleep! A tired brain is an uncooperative brain.

THE IMPORTANCE OF CLASSROOM LOGISTICS

Ask any real estate agent what are the three most important considerations when buying a new home. The reply is inevitably the same: Location! Location! Location! It is a valid point. After all, a house located next to the county dump is much less desirable than the same model located on the perimeter of the local country club. As a home buyer, you would never settle on a particular dwelling without first taking a careful look at the surroundings.

The same principle applies in the classroom. A classroom is a microcosm of a neighborhood. It contains a collection of people whose common interest in a particular subject has drawn them to the same place. Your seat in that classroom is your dwelling for the semester. Before selecting it, consider your surroundings with a critical eye. Your goal here is to find a spot that will optimize the learning experience.

Are you easily distracted? Sit in the front center of the room. With fewer students between you and the instructor, the risk of distraction is minimized. Another benefit is that the closer you are situated to the instructor, the more familiar you will become to him or her, and your visibility will encourage you to maintain a higher level of attention than you otherwise might in a less obvious locale.

Are you anxious about being called upon, perhaps fearful of the limelight that can be suddenly shown at an inopportune time? Your anxiety can be relieved by taking a seat toward the back of the room, strategically placing insulating layers of fellow students between you and the instructor. Be advised, however, that some instructors make a point of soliciting responses from those who are perched in the far reaches of the classroom as a means of keeping all class attendees alert.

Will personal needs (physical or otherwise) likely prompt you to leave the classroom while it is in session? Sit close to the door—preferably in the back if there is a rear exit—so that you can make your escape with as little notice as possible. Where such needs are foreseen, it is a good idea to let your instructor know so that your departure is not misinterpreted as lack of interest (or even worse, lack of respect).

Every neighborhood has its characters, and so too does each classroom. Over time, the profiles of your classmates emerge. As they do, determine whether they make good classroom neighbors. Are they inclined to make frequent sidebar comments? Do they sit still? Do they have annoying tics? Do they engage in activities that are unrelated to classroom discourse, such as sketching or texting? Identify the idiosyncrasies of your classmates. Determine whether their peculiarities are going to detract from your ability to concentrate on the instruction you are being given, and relocate if you need to.

Consider as well your own level of creature comfort. Temperatures in the classroom can be extreme, particularly in older buildings. They can be hot (so wear clothing that can be removed as needed in layers) or cold (bring a sweater). If dimly lit, move closer to the window. And if you can prevent it, never come to class hungry. A rumbling stomach will compete with the instructor for your attention.

HOW TO STAY FOCUSED DURING CLASS

Sit erect, don't slump! Does it sound like grade school? The physiological reason for sitting up straight is to allow the much-needed oxygen to reach the bellows of your lungs and be distributed throughout your body during lectures, especially to your brain! Learn to practice deep relaxation breathing periodically during a class lecture. It will help to wake you up and increase your blood circulation. At the same time, move in your seat if you feel sleepy. Keep eye contact with your instructors.

A good poker player is always on the lookout for another player's "tell." This is an unconscious mannerism or gesture that signals the strength of the hand he has been dealt. In the context of the classroom, teachers have tells as well. Discover them! It could be a slight change in voice inflection, a more intense gaze, or some other subtlety that indicates the point being made is an important one, and one that will likely reappear on an upcoming exam.

If the lecture you are about to receive will last more than two hours, it is a good idea to bring some form of nourishment if the teacher does not object. Not all school buildings have cafeterias and the hours may be intermittent for those that do. Bring protein bars, fruit, cheese and crackers, etc. You may want to bring some form of caffeine with you but avoid high-energy drinks so you will not be restless in your seat. Whatever food or drink you decide to carry in, be discreet in their consumption. Remember that you are attending a class lecture, not a class picnic. Chomping, slurping, belching, drooling, and so forth are out of place in citadels of learning and are a distraction to your teacher and fellow classmates.

A longer lecture will often have at least one break. Use it wisely. During breaks, walk around. Just like you are advised to stretch and walk around during a long airplane flight, do this with long classes during breaks. Some students learn to list questions on a separate piece of paper during class and then during breaks approach the teacher with a few questions. Most instructors will be complimented that you listened and have inquiries. Some will answer your questions there and others will suggest an after-class appointment so the response receives the time it warrants. It is also possible that they will gently steer you toward some of the more important data or material in their lectures as a way to help you study since you have demonstrated so much interest.

Some students choose to record all nursing lectures (again, with the teacher's permission). Much can be missed if you rely on memory alone or your notes. If you have ever watched the same movie a second time, you invariably pick up on dialogue you missed the first time. Nursing lectures are no different in that regard and their repetition can only reinforce your knowledge base.

=*FAST FACTS in a NUTSHELL*

- Prepare by reading the material to be presented in class before the class.
- Create outlines for yourself as a method to begin to absorb the information and use this outline as a format for your note taking in class.
- Choose your classroom seat with care and use every minute of class time wisely.

5

Interacting With Your Instructor

INTRODUCTION

Instructors are people, too. They have their own style of delivering information and their own standards in terms of expectations of their students. Understanding your instructor's strengths and vulnerabilities will go a long way toward a peaceful and productive coexistence.

In this chapter, you will learn:

1. What the syllabus tells you about the instructor.
2. How to accommodate your instructor's teaching style.
3. How to conduct yourself in one-on-one encounters with your instructor.

WHAT THE SYLLABUS TELLS YOU ABOUT THE INSTRUCTOR

Have you ever noticed that some instructors have a three- or four-page syllabus and others have one page, or that one instructor will take fifteen minutes to give you directions that a different instructor delivers in four minutes? Those observations can tell you a lot about your nursing instructor in terms of his or her attention to detail. If details are important to them, they should be important to you. If you pay attention to these differences, your life as a nursing student will go more smoothly.

A syllabus will often address the topic of class attendance. Nursing is a profession in which classroom attendance is usually mandatory. This often translates into penalties or rewards for consistent attendance. In fact, you usually will have a penalty for missing a nursing class. The rationale for attaching rewards to attendance is that the information delivered may not be repeated again in any forum (this is especially true for the accelerated, second-degree programs). Thus, it is vital that a nursing student attends classroom lectures. If the history major misses class and fails to learn the date of the signing of the Treaty of Versailles, his credibility as a history expert can potentially suffer. If the nursing student misses class and does not learn the standard precautions to prevent spread of infection, a patient could die as a result.

Carefully read the syllabus to ascertain what this instructor deems most important. If the psychosocial assessment is worth 20 of 100 points, note that this instructor strongly believes that students need to understand the psychosocial components of patients and disease. If proper American Psychological Association (APA) formatting on your term paper is required in the syllabus, buy the APA reference book and have a colleague familiar with this formatting proofread your term paper to avoid losing points.

HOW TO ACCOMMODATE YOUR INSTRUCTOR'S TEACHING STYLE

Some teachers will distribute either online or in a course pack (a required group of pages bought at a bookstore with vital information for the nursing class) a preclass outline to be completed before their lecture. A word to the wise: Complete this outline.

Think about it. Why would an instructor go to the trouble to read the chapter and material and then create a preclass outline? Often this outline will be your key to successful studying for this professor and will save you the trouble of creating one yourself from scratch. Other teachers do not require this level of advance preparation but will note for their classes what to read beforehand. Take your lead from your teacher.

Some professors are not born lecturers. Despite their considerable credentials, their articulation may make them hard to understand and their delivery arduous to listen to. Yes, some are BORING! Be patient with them. They are probably doing their best and often there is not an audition for the best orator when it comes to hiring nursing instructors. Consider their predicament for a moment. It is not a walk in the park to translate difficult concepts into succinct and sparkling lectures.

Other professors may continually read from their projected PowerPoint slides with very little student interaction throughout the lecture. While this teaching style is not the preference of most nursing students, try to remain alert because important information is being disseminated. Stay awake and ask questions to relieve the tedium of the class.

Finally, be on guard with those who teach nothing from the required readings. Their penchant is to ramble on about their experiences. Their past nursing adventures may be fascinating or have no coherent flow to their topic. In either case, these teachers are the ones to be careful with. You really must read the textbook to build a foundation of knowledge and ask them what specifically they would suggest that you study for their exams.

HOW TO CONDUCT YOURSELF IN ONE-ON-ONE ENCOUNTERS WITH YOUR INSTRUCTOR

Don't hesitate to make appointments with your nursing instructors. They are human even though at times it may not seem so. They once were nursing students like you and maybe not even back in the Stone Age. As with most professions, some are better than others. You will find those who are enthusiastic and glowing examples of what a nurse educator should be. You will also find people who got into nursing education and stayed with it when that may not have been their best career choice. Put your personal likes and dislikes aside and know that you can learn something from each one (even if it is what NOT to do once you become a nurse).

The field experience of your instructors will also vary. At one end of the continuum are those instructors who have acquired much in the way of direct patient care experience before they start to teach. At the other end are those who have gone into teaching and perhaps research rather early in their nursing careers. Both can offer perspectives that you can profit from. Seek out those instructors who have taken the path that you intend to traverse in the nursing profession and profit from their personal insights.

Feel free to make appointments with your teachers to discuss questions, but approach these one-on-one encounters with due respect. Don't bluntly ask, "What do I need to know for the exam?" This is like a red flag to a bull. Rather, go in with written questions that demonstrate that you have done your homework before entering your teacher's office and taking up his or her valuable time. One especially astute student suggests that questions be posed deferentially as follows: "I understand . . ., but I am still having trouble with . . . Can you help me?" The reward often is that the instructor will point you in a direction of study that will be the most profitable for you, and you will have made a good impression in return.

Don't forget a simple "thank you note" or, if you prefer, an email thanking the professor for the time taken to help you, but only if you are sincere. Those notes mean a lot to your teacher, who as we now know is only human.

FAST FACTS in a NUTSHELL

- Instructors are human, so treat them as such.
- Don't hesitate to make appointments with your nursing instructors.
- Carefully read the syllabus to ascertain what this instructor deems most important.

6

What Kind of Learner Are You?

INTRODUCTION

Although their means of categorization may differ, various studies have concluded that not all people learn the same way.

In this chapter, you will learn:

1. Strategies in building your knowledge base.
2. How you may learn best.
3. Critical thinking in the learning process.
4. Tips on test taking.
5. Coping with learning differences.

The fortune cookie was snapped in half, and out tumbled the proverb: "Tell me and I will forget; show me and I may remember; let me do it myself and I will learn." This crunchy bit of wisdom points to the fact that not all people learn the same way. The author was obviously a person who learns by doing. While he himself may not profit greatly by being told or shown, the fact is that many others can and do comprehend new information in those ways. In the course of your nursing education, you can expect to learn by being told, shown, and supervised as you eventually perform nursing procedures on your own. In the end, your own wisdom and critical thinking skills will be your best navigator of present and future learning.

STRATEGIES IN BUILDING YOUR KNOWLEDGE BASE

It is easy to categorize milk. Milk is either whole, low-fat, or nonfat. Everyone agrees with this method of labeling and understands what the labels represent. Not so with labeling learning styles. Some experts have constructed alternate models of segmenting the population in terms of how they learn. The contention of these experts is that having insight into how you most efficiently process incoming information enables you to adopt learning approaches that are a good match for you personally.

It is beyond the scope of this book to explore these varying philosophies. More pertinent to our discussion are the tools nursing students have available to them in the learning process. No one learning approach is better than another on the surface, but personal preference can lead you to adopt certain ones and reject others as you march along the educational path to your nursing license. Among the more common learning approaches employed by nursing students are:

- *Taking detailed notes in class*
Note taking keeps you focused on the lecture and can help you pick up on points that are not in the textbook.

- *Taping lectures*
Taping lectures continues to grow in popularity as a verbatim record of the lecture, but ask permission from your instructor first as lectures can be considered intellectual property.

- *Outlining textbook chapters*
Outlining synthesizes the content of what can often be a prodigious amount of reading material.

- *Reading the textbook*
In view of the density of material in most nursing books, many students recommend skimming text where possible but thoroughly reading areas that need reinforcement.

- *Viewing a live demonstration*
Seeing nursing procedures performed in action is a good complement to studying them in class.

- *Looking at an instructional video*
Videos allow for in-depth instruction through voice-overs and close-ups.

- *Practicing a skill*
Practice ensures that your conceptual grasp of the information is accurate.

- *Joining a study group*
Study groups assign topics to their members for in-depth study, and members subsequently share their work with other team members. Alternately, study groups can simply be a forum for discussion with each member responsible for his or her own study. They are not for everyone, as discussed later.

- *Finding a study partner*
Compatibility is easier to find in a study partner than a study group, but the workload is proportionately larger when only two students are involved.

- *Answering questions at the end of the textbook chapter*
Traditionally ignored if not required by the instructor, the end-of-chapter textbook questions provide a good overview of the topic.

- *Review printed lecture slides*

Printed slides can offer a synopsis of the information covered but may be insufficient unless accompanied by notes that are added by the student as the lecture progresses.

- *Discussion with instructor outside of class*

A dialogue with your instructor can plug knowledge gaps by clarifying concepts covered in class. More on this later.

HOW DO YOU LEARN BEST?

Only you know the correct response to this question. However, an informal survey of nursing students reveals some consensus as to which learning techniques work best in given situations. Their responses illustrate that learning strategies that work well in the classroom are not necessarily as valuable at the clinical site, and vice versa. Classroom learning involves the acquisition and mastering of new concepts and understanding their interrelatedness to the knowledge you already have. Clinical learning, on the other hand, involves applying your knowledge in the analysis of a patient's condition and the performance of therapeutic procedures. These two different spheres produce two different lists of preferred learning techniques as described next.

CLASSROOM Learning Techniques in Order of Preference	
1	Take detailed notes in class.
2	Read the textbook.
3	Review printed lecture slides.
4	Outline textbook chapters.
5	Tape lectures.

CLINICAL* Learning Techniques in Order of Preference

1	Practice the skill.
2	Read the textbook.
3	Look at instructional videos.
4	View a live demonstration.
5	Tape lectures.

*CLINICAL-based courses include topics such as head-to-toe assessment, vital sign procurement, hygiene and comfort, standard precautions, and other initial nursing skills.

Notice that two learning approaches appear on both the Classroom and Clinical lists. These are reading the textbook and taping the lectures. Based on our informal survey, incorporating these two strategies into your learning process will pay double dividends.

CRITICAL THINKING IN THE LEARNING PROCESS

The combination of learning techniques that work best for you will comprise your learning style. The optimal learning style is the one that will enable you to think critically as you link new concepts with those you have already mastered to expand your knowledge base. As one principle builds upon another, your critical thinking skills will be needed more and more to make sense of what you are learning. That magical moment as you experience "the light bulb being lit" will replicate itself again and again during your time in nursing school. Your need to think critically does not end with graduation. Health care and nursing is ever-evolving. Since knowledge learned today can be obsolete tomorrow, nurses must be continually prepared to learn the newest techniques and the theory behind them to provide their patients with the best care possible.

For this reason, some professors use critical thinking during their lectures. These are the teachers who might ask a complex question in class, one that requires real thinking as opposed to simple rote answers. Accurate responses will require sifting through previous knowledge, choosing what facts are most essential and applicable, and integrating different levels of information to arrive at an answer. One common forum for critical thinking is the case study. In a case study, professors provide students with a situation and its pertinent facts. Often you will be permitted to work in a group in which you and the other members collaborate in assessing the situation and determining the proper course of action to follow in resolving it.

Be grateful for these opportunities. Your interaction with your peers as you seek their perspectives and offer them your own will continue throughout your nursing career. A word of caution must be offered here, however. Sometimes students choose to spend this valuable time discussing their weekend plans or the probable questions in the exam for the next class. DON'T DO IT! Use this class time wisely. Try to associate yourself with the students who take case studies seriously, even if you need to change the group you are in.

Your entire practice as a nurse will involve working with a team of others to achieve a goal that will depend on critical thinking. If a patient starts to reach a crisis in the hospital, it takes a team to diagnose the patient, develop a plan, and implement it—often in the space of a few minutes. A successful end to such drama actually begins years earlier in the classroom, as nursing students begin to transform information into knowledge through the learning style that suits them best.

TIPS ON TEST TAKING

Nursing exam questions can be tricky. Even second-degree nursing students often have difficulty adjusting to nursing questions. They come from fields such as accounting, journalism, biology, chemistry, and many other prestigious majors. They consider themselves good readers and have been able to successfully navigate a field of study to achieve a college degree. And yet, nursing questions can initially "throw" even these accomplished students. An example of a typical nursing question would be the following:

> When assessing for a patient's popliteal pulse, the nurse is unable to palpate it.
>
> Which action by the nurse would be the best action to take next?
>
> a. Ask another nurse to assist and palpate for the pulse.
>
> b. Palpate for the pedal pulse.
>
> c. Palpate for the femoral pulse.
>
> d. Call the physician.

A knowledge of anatomy alone is not enough to arrive at the correct answer. Selecting the best response also requires a logical conclusion that builds on that knowledge of anatomy to arrive at an answer that will not necessarily be found in a textbook. The term "best response" is appropriate because nursing questions can offer more than one viable alternative in the answer bank. In the question above, a nurse calling the physician would certainly get the patient problem resolved, but that would not be the best course of action in that it would needlessly delay assistance to the patient while at the same time drawing the physician away from other patients whose needs are greater. Once again we see the importance of critical thinking by the nurse, whose day-to-day resolution of questions such as the one above plays a vital role in protecting patients' lives. By the way, the correct response to the question above is "b."

Nursing questions rarely involve a regurgitation of factual information only. Rather, they require an in-depth understanding of the topic and the ability to effectively synthesize that information in the context of a hypothetical situation. Always read nursing questions carefully. A single word within the question can have vital importance in terms of how it is answered.

Testing is a shared experience, so study groups can be helpful when you have such a large amount of information to learn in such a short time. Some students benefit from being part of a study group. Others may find it is a big waste of time. Does the study group often just become a gossip session as precious minutes tick away? Does it increase your anxiety, leaving you feel that everyone knows so much more than you? Or does it slow you down as you determine that you are much further along than other group members in your grasp of the material? To borrow the words of William Shakespeare, "To thine own self be true!" Participate in study groups or avoid them sometimes or entirely based on whatever works best for you.

Often overlooked by students is another valuable opportunity—request a meeting with your nursing professor before each exam. This system works best if you make an appointment and prepare for the meeting. Simply dropping in to ask, "What will be on the exam?" will not help your cause and may in fact alienate you from this instructor. Similarly, pose your questions in such a way as to indicate that you have at least tried to do your part in the learning process. The most successful students go to these meetings with questions such as, "I understand that there are three different types of kidney failure and that the most common is prerenal. I am still having trouble understanding intrarenal failure. Could you help me understand it better?" Most instructors respect this type of question and will be happy to explain their material to you.

Test anxiety has been around since Adam and Eve faced the apple. Basically, it involves one's own sympathetic nervous system overreacting to a stimulus like an exam and preventing one from thinking clearly in answering questions to the best of his or her ability. Sometimes, one bad experience in the past, like forgetting to study a whole section and being tested on it, or doing poorly and being embarrassed by someone, will set up a reaction to future exams that will interfere with your performance. If this sounds like you, there is help. Learn simple relaxation techniques that you can use before, during, and after exam situations. Exercise regularly, get enough sleep the night before the exam, don't drink too much caffeine (the perfect trigger for excess sympathetic nervous stimulation and anxiety), and practice slow deep breathing. Relaxation breathing can be as simple as breathing in to the count of 4 and breathing out to the count of 5. Practice before the exam at home, in the car, and during the exam if you feel yourself getting too anxious.

Many nursing professors will have an exam review session sometime after the exam. Take advantage of these sessions and use them for their intended purpose. This is not the time to argue with the professor for an additional point or two. Most professors use nursing questions that have been already been tested for validity and reliability. Pay attention to your mistakes. Do you find that if you changed an answer, that the original answer was correct? Did you rush through the exam, making simple mistakes? The purpose of an exam review is for learners to discover and subsequently remedy their pattern of mistakes and, more importantly, to learn the correct information. Failing to really understand a principle or a piece of knowledge could result in harm to a patient in the future.

Finally, don't exaggerate the ultimate importance of grades. Sure, there will be fellow students, parents, spouses, and even nursing faculty who will espouse the merits of achieving all As. Listen politely, but the fact is that getting straight As within a nursing curriculum is not at all easy. So, don't die trying. Good grades in lieu of great ones will do just fine when it is time to look for a nursing position, as the better recruiters evaluate the whole person, not just the GPA.

In nursing, test taking involves more than simply getting your degree. As a nursing student, you will one day face the NCLEX® (National Council Licensure Examination for Registered Nurses)—the nursing board exam of the state that you intend to be licensed in. Even if you were to earn your nursing degree, you cannot practice as a registered nurse unless you pass the nursing board exam! A word to the wise: Don't wait until 3 months before you plan to take the nursing board exam to practice answering the type of questions you are going to encounter. Begin preparing for the board exam right from the start. Begin during your first semester by addressing those "extra practice" questions supplied by most nursing texts. The more exposure you have to how the threads of nursing concepts can be woven into questions, the more adept you will be at answering them correctly when acquisition of your license depends on it. The NCLEX will be covered in more detail later in the book.

COPING WITH LEARNING DIFFERENCES

Mike entered college immediately after high school as a science major (he thought he might be a chiropractor). He averaged two to three science courses each semester and his grades were mostly high Cs, Bs, and some As. After the fall sophomore semester, he decided to go to nursing school. After his second semester of nursing school, he was in academic jeopardy. He was below the minimum grade point average of 77 for his coursework. He discussed this with his parents and described his difficulty, which centered around "reading the nursing questions." His parents consulted a neuropsychologist for testing, which revealed that Mike was dyslexic. As a result of this diagnosis Mike qualified for more time in all tests, which greatly improved his success in completing nursing exams—and in his grades. In times past someone may have advised Mike that he was just not "cut out" for nursing. Thankfully, research has shown that some exceptionally intelligent students struggle with their reading because they process information differently. With proper accommodation, students with learning differences can achieve and in fact excel academically.

Section 504 of the federal Rehabilitation Act of 1973 and the Individuals with Disabilities Education Act of 2004 (IDEA) allow each nursing student under the age of 22 with the appropriate documentation to have certain accommodations when tested while attending an institution that receives federal funds. Even institutions that do not fall into this category are usually more than willing to extend accommodations where the need has been formally established.

Although the Individualized Education Plan (IEP) primarily protects the interests of special need learners only through high school, their content may continue to apply until the learning disabled student reaches age 22. Most post–high school centers of learning have policies and procedures for students who require accommodations to be successful in the classroom. These include but are not limited to the following:

- Academic coaching
- Alternative test-taking arrangements
- Priority registration
- Note-taking support
- Study skills tutoring
- Alternate formatting assistance (e.g., Recordings for the Blind)
- Adaptive technology
- Referrals for learning disabilities testing
- More time for exam testing

To qualify for any accommodations, you will be required to provide recent and appropriate documentation prepared by a licensed professional (usually a psychologist) to the specific office in your school that coordinates these services. Check with your school regarding the particulars.

Special need students who are entitled to things like extra time in taking exams and private alternate testing may hesitate to inform their instructors of this fact. They are embarrassed by the possibility of being perceived as different by teachers and fellow classmates. If you are a special need student with a documented learning difference diagnosis, don't let your vanity foolishly deny you what is rightfully yours for the asking. And once you are approved for accommodations, make sure that you use them! You are just as "smart" as any other student in your nursing class (perhaps even smarter). Your brain processes information in a way where getting a few more minutes to read a question or taking your exam in a private testing room will elevate your performance on the exam to the best it can be. The NCLEX state licensing board exam allows accommodations for testing as long as one has the appropriate documentation.

Learning differences can be subtle. You can be highly articulate and still be challenged by reading and writing. If you even suspect that you have a learning difference, it is worth being tested now by a psychologist to determine if you are indeed affected. As already mentioned, nursing exams are tough with difficult language and high expectations. It may save you a lot of time, hardship, and money to identify and seek accommodations for a learning difference before your education program commences.

FAST FACTS in a NUTSHELL

- Optimal learning strategies in nursing can vary from person to person and from classroom to clinical site.
- Critical thinking is a vital part of the learning process.
- Students with learning disabilities should not hesitate to request accommodations from their instructors.

7

The Digital World of Nursing Education

INTRODUCTION

The application of technology to education has led to innovations that perhaps were not even in existence when your teacher was a nursing student. This chapter highlights some that quickly have become incorporated into nursing education.

In this chapter, you will learn:

1. The proper placement of patient simulation in a nursing curriculum.
2. The growth of online coursework.
3. The practical value of digital devices to a nursing student.

THE PROPER PLACEMENT OF PATIENT SIMULATION IN A NURSING CURRICULUM

Remember when you went through the process of getting a driver's license? You needed to read the driver's manual provided by your state's department of transportation to know what to do once you got out on the road. But mastering the content of the driver's manual was not enough to merit driving privileges. You also had to demonstrate your driving proficiency by passing a road test. Chances are that this test was done with the careful oversight of a state employee and on a dedicated course that was free of traffic and pedestrians. While you may not have thought about it at the time, your road test was a simulation of obstacles and situations you would encounter once on a real road.

Simulation creates an experience that represents reality, mimicking real life (Reilly & Oermann, 1992). Applied to nursing education, simulation attempts to create a hypothetical patient care environment within which nursing students can safely operate before moving on to an actual patient care setting. Although the subject of much attention in current nursing programs, simulation in nursing has been around since Florence Nightingale's day. When Florence demonstrated to her charges the proper methodology for preventing infection, she was using simulation. As described later, today's nursing students receive simulated experience in varying ways ranging from instructor demonstration to hands-on treatment of robotic figures serving as patients.

Simulation allows the nursing student to get preliminary exposure to the performance of a procedure or skill without the anxiety that would normally accompany the same exercise in a real-life scenario. In a simulation, no harm will come to a patient if the student nurse fails to execute a process correctly. Every mistake is reversible because the instructor controls the outcome. Simulation can be as simple as using case studies (scenarios in a written format that allow the nursing student group to use team skills to formulate a treatment plan for the client). Simulation also occurs when the nursing instructor demonstrates in a classroom a procedure such as how to assess lung sounds.

At the more advanced level, there is mannequin-based simulation where a replica of a human patient is used to demonstrate a skill such as transferring a person from a bed to a chair. Sometimes in simulation human actors are used to allow the students to talk with a person posing as a patient as they practice interviewing skills. Students can practice simulation with each other to accomplish this goal also.

You may hear the word "fidelity" associated with simulation. Fidelity indicates the degree of realism achieved by the simulation. For example, two nursing instructors demonstrating a patient interview for a group of nursing students may serve the purpose of simulation but the reality achieved is quite limited. The student knows that the nursing instructors are the actors. Fidelity is particularly important as it relates to mannequins. Low fidelity would describe mannequins that are just plastic models, providing no interaction but allowing skill demonstration of such things as urinary catheterization or wound dressing change. High fidelity mannequins are more realistic in that they can portray bowel, breath, and heart sounds along with changing blood pressure, respiratory, and heart rates. Some are remotely controlled by a computer in another room, and physiological changes can occur instantly. These physiological changes can be assessed by the student nurses as they count the radial pulse or as the vital signs appear on a screen in the room.

Despite continued advances in simulation technology, nothing can replicate the experience of talking with and caring for the human being you encounter in the clinical setting. Why? Imagine a video of the ocean beach. One hears the sound of the crashing waves on the shore and sees the shimmering sun reflecting off the mirror of the water as the camera follows the flight of a seagull soaring over the tranquil scene. If that experience can be fully captured on a video, why would so many people invest their time and money traveling to the ocean's coast each year just to sit on a beach? Obviously, the video cannot fully convey what it is like to really be at the beach—the aroma of the ocean, the warmth of the sand, and so on. Similarly, no nursing lab simulation can ever fully acquaint you with the connection you will feel toward your patient and the connection that your patient will feel toward you. Whether the patient care activity is treating, educating, bathing, or simply soothing the soul, it is the interpersonal aspect that raises the healing art of nursing to its highest form.

As a result, you want to question in detail exactly how your nursing program employs simulation. While simulation is a wonderful adjunct to your learning, be careful that it is not used to significantly reduce the more valuable component of clinical time (time working with real patients) that you are entitled to. Some schools may try to sell the notion that a day in the "sim lab" can effectively reproduce the same challenges that you would face as a nurse in a real-life hospital unit. Be very wary of these claims! If you want to graduate with a sense of confidence in your nursing skills, you need to take care of real patients as a nursing student.

THE GROWTH OF ONLINE COURSEWORK

The demand for online programs has increased over the past ten to fifteen years. It is easy to understand why. In a time-constrained world, online courses can be much more convenient for student and instructor alike.

The faculty role in online instruction is more of a coach and mentor as opposed to the traditional lecturer role. Meetings are asynchronous, which means that postings of comments based on required readings or previous work will be at different intervals—not at the same time, as in a person-to-person classroom. There are some classes where there is some real-time interaction, but the majority of classes are not interactive.

Learning resources are more flexible. There will be I-units, smartphones, and all manners of hand-held devices that will render knowledge acquisition more mobile and flexible.

Assessments and discussion boards are continuous, with group projects and exams that occur throughout the course.

Be prepared to participate three to five times a week with your online classroom. Most people questioned find online courses may actually require more work than that of the traditional classroom.

Online learners are necessarily more participative. Online discussions require previous reading and analysis, and then individual postings. There is no sitting in the back of the room and avoiding eye contact with the teacher. Are you a self-motivator? Do you enjoy working at your own pace and on your own timetable? Or do you work better with a class-mate to encourage you and when interacting with fellow classmates about assignments, etc.? These are all consider-ations you must weigh before you enroll in an online course.

To the extent they are offered in nursing programs, online courses may represent a viable alternative in learning nursing theory and in fulfilling elective course requirements that are outside of the nursing curriculum. Obviously, they are by their nature incompatible with nursing education needs warranting instructor demonstration or student hands-on practice.

THE PRACTICAL VALUE OF DIGITAL DEVICES TO A NURSING STUDENT

The recent emergence and relative value of electronic devices to record lectures, take notes, retrieve information, and com-municate with peers and instructors have created a learning experience with many more options.

Most nursing instructors have become accustomed to beginning a lecture with a sea of recording devices strewn in front of them. As they stand at a podium or travel through-out the classroom, tiny recording devices are capturing their voices and their thoughts. It can give a lecturer pause prior to offering some of the usual commentary that many seasoned professors sprinkle throughout their lectures for the sake of humor or stimulation. While entertaining in the moment, they may not be suitable for posterity. Remember to ask permission to record the instructor's lectures before you attempt to carry away your instructor's work on a recording device. With that courtesy extended, most instructors will be agreeable with your recording request.

With Internet access, smartphones represent a fast and effective way to obtain information. A discussion or disagreement about the latest guidelines for mammograms can be quickly settled by allowing students to "Google" this information. Just be confident in the legitimacy of the information source you access before incorporating it in your patient care.

Personal digital assistants (PDAs) have also emerged as a vital technical tool for nurses, but their applicability to the clinical site is much greater than it is in the classroom. The usefulness of PDAs in clinical situations will be covered in Part III.

So what is the bottom line regarding student use of digital devices? Informal observation indicates that students find smartphone apps convenient for clinical site uses such as looking up medications, finding patient diagnosis descriptions, and defining technical terms. On the other hand, students prefer books to electronic resources for studying, preparing nursing journal entries developing nursing care plans, and writing research papers.

FAST FACTS in a NUTSHELL

- Simulation is an important educational tool that can range from basic skill demonstration to computer-driven patient mannequins.
- Simulation should not be considered as a replacement for clinical time with real patients.
- One of the most useful electronic devices to bring into the classroom is a recording device.

In Student Nurses' Own Words . . .

"Reading prior to class was super helpful, not just because you can answer questions but you also understand the material a whole lot better. Exams are 50% harder than a normal college exam. The 'A' student can easily become a 'C' student and still do just as well in the long run with a bunch more practice in the application of the material. Some professors will be more helpful than others. It is not the end of the world if you have a bad meeting with one professor."

"Keep up with your class work! Do all the work and then some extra so you can learn all you can. Join a study group if that helps you to learn better, but study groups are not for everyone."

"Change your opinion of what is a good grade or you will be disappointed. Get to know the faculty."

"It was very helpful to record lectures. Listening to them later, you will often hear things you may have missed while taking notes. Be sure to read the textbook to give your understanding clarity."

"Be prepared for a lot of work—it is well worth it."

"Professors' lectures are a good information resource since it is not always possible to read every page of the text. Use the textbook to clarify and supplement the information you receive in lectures."

"Your professors want you to succeed, so use them. Come to class all of the time. Give yourself plenty of time to study."

"Do as much of the readings before class as possible. Look up words and topics you hear a lot—they'll keep coming back. Do the end of chapter questions in the text. Ask for help and ask questions. Use your teacher's knowledge and willingness to teach you."

"It is important to study and really learn the information because you are dealing with real people and their lives!"

"Record the lectures. You don't realize how much you miss in a lecture until you hear it for a second time. It is helpful to skim the text before class. Don't study to memorize—study to understand! Test questions often have more than one right answer, and you will need to choose the best one."

"Definitely don't cram. Review for tests at least a couple of days early."

"Take really good notes and highlight any point that the teacher says is important as it will most likely be on the test."

"While it is important to understand the content of printed slides, you should also read the text for knowledge and advancement."

"I found using a recorder very helpful. In addition, I recommend taking actual notes instead of relying on printed slides. This way you can go back and listen to the recording and *rewrite your notes. In terms of studying, I would definitely start early on before the exam, not two days before."*

"Don't be afraid to ask questions. Someone else will have that same question. Practice NCLEX® questions on sites complementing the textbook (chapters). Find out what works best for you—study groups or studying alone. For term papers, write a rough draft and ask for suggestions for improvement before finishing, since all professors grade papers differently. Look at your notes and study every day, since you will forget the first lecture by the time you are tested on it. Readings are overwhelming. Skim the titles and headings and if you don't understand something in class, then read that section of the book. Try not to take courses you know will be difficult (such as microbiology and pathophysiology) at the same time if at all possible. Summer is a good time to take a difficult course."

"I went from an 'A' student in my general education classes to a 'C' student in my nursing classes before I learned how to succeed. Stay on top of the readings, which are a lot but really do supplement what is learned in class. Focus on application of the information—don't memorize every last detail."

"Pay attention in class. It's only a few hours out of your life, so give it your best shot. Get feedback from the professor on a draft of your term paper so you know you are on the right track. Read exam questions very carefully. Sometimes you will miss the importance of words like 'not' and 'except.'"

"Recorders are helpful when you have teachers who talk fast or are covering a hard topic. Listening to the lecture later will help clarify your notes. Teachers like when you use their office hours to ask questions. It shows you are interested in the material and want to succeed in nursing."

"Be realistic is setting your goals. Are you really going to get all of that work done in one night? Get two readers for your term paper, since one teacher's 'C' can be another teacher's 'A.'"

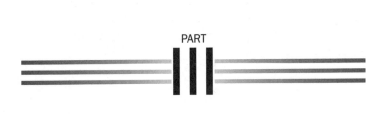

PART

III

Success at the Clinical Site

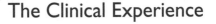

8

The Clinical Experience

INTRODUCTION

Today's nurse is in constant motion, shuttling back and forth between the technical aspects of nursing practice and the human aspects of nursing care. There are few other professions that require their practitioners to be so adept in so many different ways. As a nurse, you can treat, educate, console, bathe, and medicate a patient all within the same day. The clinical component of your nursing program will begin to acquaint you with the need to be multidimensional. You can get off to a good start by knowing how to conduct yourself as a student who has now crossed the threshold into the real world of nursing.

In this chapter, you will learn:

1. Personal prerequisites for success at the clinical site.
2. Rules of the road as a new health care provider.
3. Patient confidentiality.

Jean stopped by the clinical instructor's office a week before her first clinical rotation. She had scored well in her exams but just needed some reassurance before she stepped onto a nursing floor. "If I do well in my nursing class work, I will do well in my clinical rotation—right?"

The answer is—maybe. Obviously there is a strong correlation between good classroom performance and good clinical performance. You need to have laid the conceptual groundwork that your clinical experience seeks to build on. But there are differences worth noting between classrooms and clinical that can be problematic to some "A" students and a confidence booster to their less accomplished counterparts.

Classroom exams tap the brain's memory and learning skills. Many nursing students have the innate ability to be "good test takers." They have the cognitive ability to easily digest classroom content and commit it to memory. Clinical skills, however, are very different. While they certainly depend on your class work as a foundation, they also require superior analytical aptitude, psychomotor abilities, and emotional intelligence.

In the clinical education setting, students need to apply classroom knowledge to "real world" situations. The hypothetical congestive heart failure patient you studied in the classroom is now right in front of you and not able to breathe! Are you able to assess and implement life-saving strategies immediately, which include recognizing the seriousness of the situation and informing your instructor and the primary nurse? Sometimes students may receive As on nursing exams but do not recognize the "real world" situation at hand, resulting in delay in procuring assistance for the patient.

Clinical competence also requires the psychomotor skills of assessment, bathing, performing complex nursing procedures, supervising intravenous therapies, etc. Book knowledge will translate into performance only with experience, and the duration of that learning curve will vary from one individual to another as they are exposed to different patient situations.

Last, there is the aspect of emotional intelligence, popularized by Daniel Goleman and referenced in Part I of this book. To reiterate, emotional intelligence can be loosely described as the ability of an individual to accurately discern the feelings of another in the course of an encounter. As a nurse, you will find that much of what is wrong or worrying a patient can be unspoken. Patients often do not know what to say to the health care professionals. They may actually be fearful to tell them about a certain pain. Will they keep me in the hospital if I tell them I felt faint when I first got up this morning? It takes emotional intelligence on the nurse's part to recognize and seize upon those subtle cues offered by a patient as to what is really wrong, and to know what to say and how to say it in response.

So, despite its importance, classroom knowledge facilitates but does not always guarantee clinical success.

PERSONAL PREREQUISITES FOR SUCCESS AT THE CLINICAL SITE

Clinical courses will usually take place at hospitals, community health centers, skilled and assisted nursing agencies, nursing home-care agencies, schools, and outpatient facilities. These organizations have agreements with the nursing schools allowing students to participate in the care of their clients, patients, and residents. While clinical education is a logical progression from classroom education, it does not happen automatically.

Many nursing programs have requirements called technical standards that must first be met by nursing students in order to qualify for enrollment in a clinical nursing course. These requirements usually state that the student must meet the technical standards alone or with "reasonable" accommodations. Reasonable accommodations are usually decided upon by the school's office of disabilities and the nursing department in tandem. The language of these requirements usually reads like this:

Technical Standards for Clinical Education Eligibility

All students must be able to demonstrate that they have the ability to perform these skills with minimal assistance:

General abilities: Use of senses of vision, touch, hearing, smell must by integrated so the student can assess patients.

Social skills: Integrity, concern for others, compassion, being flexible in a changing environment, and managing very stressful situations.

Psychomotor skills: Sit, stand, walk, move equipment or person, reach, record, legibly document, palpate, manipulate small equipment pieces like blood pressure equipment, identify colors and color changes.

Ability to hear and receive directions: Respond to team members verbally and in written formats, communicate on the spot to patients, students, team members, etc.

Maintain self-care: Good health, arrange self transportation, appropriate control of affective behaviors like emotions, physical and mental health.

Be aware that you may be required to sign a statement acknowledging your informed consent to comply with standards as noted above in order to continue in a nursing program.

Additional Prerequisites

Nursing students will need to undergo their own *physical exam*. Included in a physical exam will be tuberculosis testing, eye examination, evidence of immunity to measles, mumps, rubeola, rubella, polio, tetanus, diphtheria, hepatitis B, and varicella.

Substance abuse is yet another area for which student nurses must receive testing. A designated time and place for *drug testing* will be assigned to each student. Some of the substances that the test will screen for will be amphetamines, barbiturates, benzodiazepines, cannabinoids, cocaine, opiates, and alcohol. It is advisable to inform the director of nursing if you are prescribed a drug that may appear in any of these screens. You may be required to submit to substance abuse testing yearly and a positive test result can lead to dismissal from the nursing program.

It is not uncommon for nursing programs to mandate that their students receive *cardiopulmonary resuscitation (CPR) certification* in life support before entering a clinical area. Usually students procure that certification independently through the American Heart Association or the American Red Cross. Look online to find clear, detailed steps to take in achieving this goal. Caution! Don't wait until a week or two before the clinical begins. CPR courses may only be offered locally at certain times and are usually preceded by online exams that must first be passed before moving on to class sessions.

In addition to personal *health insurance*, nursing students are required to have their own individual *malpractice insurance*. Many purchase the latter through coverages available online. Google nursing student malpractice insurance; applications can be completed online. It is relatively cheap—often under $50 per year.

Finally, nursing students about to begin working with patients will need appropriate *legal clearances*. Most facilities that host clinicals require evidence that each student has completed a criminal background check (obtained from the state and sometimes the FBI) and has received child abuse history clearance prior to entry into the program or the first clinical course. Some states require students to also complete an elder abuse history clearance form. If a student's criminal history reveals even a misdemeanor such as shoplifting, the clinical site has the option of denying that student access. This presents a huge problem for the nursing student. A student cannot successfully complete a nursing program without access and work time at a clinical site! The clinical host organization has the right to examine the student's record and decide, based on the incident, if that student will be able to enter their doors. This being the case, many schools now are requiring these clearances *before* acceptance into the nursing program. Successfully passing this milestone does not mean that you are out of the woods. Usually you are required to repeat these clearances every year in the nursing program. State boards of nursing (agencies that regulate the practice of nursing) may refuse applications for professional nursing licensure if the applicant "has been convicted, or has pleaded guilty, or entered a plea of nolo contendere, or has been found guilty by a judge or jury, of a felony or a crime of moral turpitude, or has received probation without verdict, disposition in lieu of trial" (National Council of State Boards of Nursing, 2011). This is true even if the crime was not related to the practice of nursing or not committed while in the practice of nursing. Be forewarned!

Take all of these requirements seriously. Nursing faculties are very astute and each student's profile will be scrutinized for all required certifications and clearances prior to their first day at a clinical site.

RULES OF THE ROAD AS A NEW
HEALTH CARE PROVIDER

You finally have reached the stage in your nursing program that you have worked so hard to achieve. The anatomy, physiology, chemistry, pathology, psychology, and sociology courses have all led you to this moment—your first clinical rotation as a student nurse. What can you expect? Are you nervous? Do you feel that despite your best efforts in preparation, you really don't know enough to render care to another human being?

Don't worry. What you are feeling is normal. Most students confess to being very nervous about clinical and feeling unprepared. In truth, this is usually a good sign since it marks you as a person who appreciates the seriousness of the responsibility you have as you enter a patient's room. You will be among five to ten students assigned to one clinical instructor. That clinical instructor will begin the course by giving you an "orientation day." Pay attention! You need to know the rules of the road for each instructor and each clinical facility. The rules will change with each new rotation, but safety is always at the top of the priority list as it relates to both you and each person whom you will encounter in the course of your clinical experience.

Clinical instructions will likely be online. Print a copy and keep it with you at all times. You do not want to violate any of the orientation or safety rules. Included in your clinical orientation will be information on safety, absence policy, dress code, facility requirements, instructor requirements, code of conduct, grading, etc. Ask any questions you may have on the first day so that your uncertainty about the rules does not lead to an unintended consequence. Be assured that any question that you may have is one that your peers have themselves or will benefit from by knowing the answer.

You may want to do a practice run before your first clinical day. Clinical sites are often spread over a large radius from your school of nursing in order to provide the very best experiences possible for you. Don't start off on the wrong foot with your instructor by being late on your first clinical day. Take a practice run a day or two before so you know where you are going and where to park (if driving). Don't forget to factor in any traffic or pedestrian congestion that may be occurring at the time you will be heading to a new clinical site for the first time. Carpool when possible to reduce expense and to receive the spiritual lift that can only come from those who are sharing your experience.

Once on-site, let your instructor get to know you. As one former student stated to a new nursing group, "Don't hide from your instructor during clinical!" Opinions will circulate regarding which instructor is "good," "tough," "mean," "easy," and so on. It is in your best interest to ignore these comments, just as you would expect your clinical instructor not to prejudge you based on the comments of other instructors. Give every instructor a fair chance and then judge his or her performance for yourself. Ask pertinent questions of your instructor but do your own preparation as well. Try to investigate and find answers yourself before asking the instructor. Statements like, "Last night I looked up information about nasogastric tubes but I still have questions about them" will go much further than just asking the instructor to explain nasogastric tubes. Remember you will need clinical instructors to write letters of recommendation for you when you are ready to enter the job market. Most employers place more weight on clinical instructors' reference letters than the classroom instructors' letters because, as previously noted, the skills and attributes required for clinical are different from those of the classroom.

An important aspect of each clinical rotation is your ability to be a team player. How well do you cooperate with your fellow students? Do you help them when you are finished with your own work? Do you assist the employees on the facility unit with other work you are capable of performing if needed? A task as simple as going to pharmacy to pick up a needed medicine for a patient will provide opportunity for learning and earn much goodwill from the nursing staff. Take advantage of every learning opportunity and volunteer for all missions or requests. Remember that nurses are observing you at clinical and often will mention to their nurse managers the names of students who impressed them. Such informal recommendations are extremely helpful if you ultimately decide to apply for positions on their units after graduation. This characteristic of going beyond what is expected (while remaining within the scope of your nursing student role) will be what your clinical instructor is watching for, and what prospective employers want to know about.

Your primary focus, however, remains your own assignment. Any change of any kind that you notice in your client or patient should be reported to a nurse or instructor immediately. You are not expected at your level to know what to do in emergency or deteriorating health conditions, but you are expected to know when and how to report those changes to the appropriate health care person.

Clinical nursing sites are areas where you may benefit from using your own personal digital device—smartphone, etc. Always get clearance from the instructor before using your smartphone in the clinical area. Applications from online sources for a drug guide, medical dictionary, or lab and diagnostics values are often available in bundles. Some students prefer to purchase books on these topics. Whatever the policy of your school and whatever your own personal preference may be, note that you will be required to use these types of information sources.

You really do not need to bring much to the clinical site beyond your own rested brain. It is, nonetheless, a good idea to ask upperclassmen what personal tools of the trade (uniform, stethoscope, etc.) they found the most useful when they went through clinical, and find out where they obtained these items. This information will allow you to confine your own purchases to what you truly need for clinical in a particular place.

Try to enjoy your clinical rotations despite your normal apprehension. Each rotation is different and your clinical instructor can make a big difference in the end result of your experience. Some clinical instructors are well-seasoned, and base their instruction and guidance on their "real world" work experiences as a nurse in an acute care facility or outpatient organization. There are, however, instances where your clinical instructors may be new to this role or lack their own self-confidence. Sometimes they also have not had much "real world" experience upon which to base their expectations of you. If you find yourself in this situation, try to learn from others at the clinical site. If, however, you believe that the educational value of your experience is compromised by your instructor's inadequacy, you may need to communicate this information to this instructor's coordinator or level leader. Do this reporting anonymously if you feel this is in your best interest, and by all means make sure you have your facts straight as to why your clinical experience was unsuccessful. Criticisms lacking in substance will be ignored.

Most often, your clinical experience will be a positive one, as echoed in the sentiments of one nursing student's journal as she approached graduation: "I feel as though this week was a successful week for me. I really enjoyed the fact that I'm advancing further from student nurse and more towards the actual role of the nurse in a real-world setting." This journal entry was recorded after her fourth week on a medical-surgical clinical unit. You, too, will begin to recognize your own personal progress after a certain number of clinicals and begin to develop an appreciation of the fact that nursing is both a science and an art.

PATIENT CONFIDENTIALITY

Confidentiality is one of the first concepts you must master as a student and then as a professional nurse. It is so important that the U.S. Congress passed the Health Insurance Portability and Accountablity Act (HIPAA) in 2003 to protect patient information from unwarranted disclosure. In obtaining your own medical care, you have signed paperwork acknowledging your receipt of your health care providers' privacy policy and authorizing them to use your information only for its intended purpose. There are civil and criminal consequences for persons who violate HIPAA. Even the accidental release of protected health information about a client can result in a fine. Gaining access to patient information under false pretense can result in a five-year jail sentence and a $100,000 fine. Few health care providers would knowingly risk these consequences but, unfortunately, lack of awareness about the ramifications of HIPAA may result in dire professional consequences.

The confidentiality of patient information extends to all information about patients, whether written on paper, saved on a computer, or spoken aloud. It includes diagnosis, treatment plan, past health condition, and payment information. If these data are so sensitive, when are you entitled to see it or share it? One health care facility gives this advice: If you are in doubt about a breach of confidentiality as you encounter or disseminate patient information in the course of your work, simply ask yourself whether the receipt or disclosure of patient information is reasonable and necessary in the discharge of nursing accountabilities.

How does this translate to your daily activities as a student nurse? Use prudence and common sense. For instance, when using a computer to distribute medication to your client, turn the screen off or minimize it if not directly in front of the screen. Keep your notes about the patient in your pocket and hidden, including in your dorm room. When possible, use initials for patients on all materials, not full names. Never put patient medical information in the regular trash; most facilities have a special container where this will be shredded later in the day. Refrain from discussing patient information at lunch in the cafeteria or on the elevator, for there are always listening ears. Speak softly in the hallways. Don't call out and please do not use intercom systems to divulge patient-identifiable information.

Any questions or confusion, or simply a need for confirmation about HIPAA's impact on your practice should be addressed to your instructor. There is no faster method to lose your ability to continue in your chosen career as a significant HIPAA violation.

FAST FACTS in a NUTSHELL

- Pay close attention to all prerequisites noted for entry into nursing and clinical.
- Be awake on orientation day for each new clinical and abide by the "rules of the road" for each clinical rotation.
- Remember you will need letters of recommendation from several clinical instructors to satisfy prospective employers. Being polite in asking for them can help your cause.
- You are being observed by the nursing staff as well as instructors during each clinical experience. Act accordingly.
- The confidentiality of patient information is paramount at all times.

Once On-Site

INTRODUCTION

You will be greeted with multiple stimuli as you walk into your first clinical site. Whether it is a community health center, an acute care hospital, or any health care setting in between, each can offer a true learning experience. There are simple steps that you can take to ensure that your clinical experiences will be fulfilling ones that draw you ever closer to a new career as a registered nurse.

In this chapter, you will learn:

1. How to interact with on-site staff.
2. How to protect your own health.
3. To touch a stranger.

Christine had looked forward to this day for a long time. She had paid careful attention to the instruction in anticipation of the big event, especially the part about the proper way to pack a parachute. And now, with her chute strapped to her back as the plane raced down the runway, she knew that this first skydive would be the culmination of her hard work. With her heart racing with the roar of the engine, she could not help asking herself—was she really ready?

Christine was as ready as you will be to parachute into your first clinical day. Perhaps there is a strange feeling that takes hold as you walk into your first client's room, as you realize in a panic that you have no idea what to say to the person you will be caring for. Don't worry—just be yourself. As you introduce yourself and inform the client/resident/patient about your purpose at that moment, you will begin to relax. A simple script like, "Hi, Mrs. Smith, I am a student nurse from XYZ School and will be assisting the nurse to care for you today" will suffice. That simple statement allows the patient to know who you are. It reinforces the fact that the nurse is in charge and clarifies your role as that of a learner.

HOW TO INTERACT WITH ON-SITE STAFF

Think of the on-site staff as being like a baseball team. A baseball team puts nine members in the field. A pitcher, a catcher, the infielders, and the outfielders take their designated positions, ready to perform when circumstances require their involvement. Each is indispensable. Could the team be successful without the center fielder? And what about the pitcher? The game cannot proceed until the pitcher throws the ball. And what about the catcher? Who would throw the ball back to the pitcher if there was no catcher? You get the idea. The same dynamic is true for a nursing team in any facility. The acute care hospital unit will have a nurse manager, nursing assistants, registered and possibly practical nurses, respiratory therapists, physical therapists, speech therapists, pharmacists, unit secretaries, and physicians, among others. One of your most important goals for each clinical experience will be to observe each team member's role and function. The following table gives a brief description of each aforementioned hospital team member's role:

Nurse manager	Registered nurse who is responsible 24/7 for the staff and the health of the unit's clients/patients
Nursing assistants (patient care technicians, student nurse externs, nurse aides)	Usually unlicensed personnel who perform a large portion of the physical care and needed tasks for the health and welfare of patients
Registered nurses (RNs)	Licensed personnel who are responsible for the overall welfare of their individual patients/clients. They administer medication, assess the patient, and determine if the plan of care is therapeutic
Practical nurses (LPNs)	Licensed personnel who report to a registered nurse. They are usually employed in skilled nursing facilities and are responsible for medication administration and co-assessment of clients/patients with the RN
Respiratory therapists	Licensed personnel who are chiefly responsible for the respiratory health of patients. They administer respiratory treatments, manage ventilators, and assess patients' respiratory status
Physical therapists	Licensed personnel who assist patients and clients to maintain and regain range of motion activities and increased mobility
Speech therapists	Licensed personnel who assist patients to regain swallowing and speech functions
Pharmacists	Licensed personnel who manage drug dispensing and perform overviews of the appropriateness of medications ordered
Unit secretaries	Assist nurses to maintain function and order in the busy world of hospital units, skilled nursing facility units, and other areas
Physicians	Licensed personnel who are responsible for the medical management of patients/clients. Nurses and physicians work together as a team and have much interaction

As you are (or perhaps are not) introduced to the staff of the facility, take note of the reception you receive. Some facility staff members express kindness and immediately exude a sense of welcome for student nurses. Others give off somewhat negative nonverbal "greetings" and just about mumble a hello. These are all important data to note. Plan your future interactions with the staff accordingly. Remember, the workers you are placed alongside of may not have been asked to help students and may view your appearance as just more work for them. This is certainly not the majority opinion or response but it does exist out there so be forewarned. In those relatively unfortunate instances, don't catastrophize about your future in nursing based on one or two nurses' less-than-cordial receptions. Just take it in stride and work hard, look up information on your own, ask questions of your instructor and nurse prudently, and help out all of the staff at each facility. Comments addressed to receptive nurses that exhibit your sincere desire to learn go a long way. Say something like, "I am eager to learn as much as I can here; I would love to watch you and if possible help out in any nursing procedure you will be doing." The result is often a call from your assigned nurse to watch or assist as they discharge their accountabilities. Make the most of these opportunities.

At the same time, never perform any task unsupervised if you are not sure of what you are doing. Don't just wing it! Your winging could cause irreparable harm to a human being.

Speak to all staff members, no matter what their title, in a respectful manner. You are on their turf! You are a guest in their house. Act accordingly. A simple introduction to the patient care tech caring for your patient is a courtesy you should extend. Say something like this: "Hi, I am Joe from ABC University and am caring for Ms. Smith in Room 324. I will be giving her medications, completing her hygiene, making her bed, walking her in the hallway and performing any other nursing task, and documenting all of the care. If there is anything I can do for you, just let me know." Your voluntary overture will ensure clear communication and cooperation from members of the team.

Help all of your fellow students daily. You may have all of your work done on schedule and have time to sit and surf the Internet until the shift ends, but next week you may be the one bombarded with patient care needs and will want a peer to assist you. *Teamwork* is the name of the game in nursing. No one is an island and no one can effectively work in isolation. It requires the efforts of a myriad of folks to properly care for each individual.

HOW TO PROTECT YOUR OWN HEALTH

You are caring for sick people of all races, creeds, and countries. Remember that many diseases are contagious and transferable. With simple and consistent strategies, your chances of getting ill yourself at a facility are minimal.

There is a policy that all health care facilities use called Standard Precautions. These precautions are constantly updated by the Centers for Disease Control and Prevention (CDC) and are mandated to be taught and re-taught yearly. Basically, Standard Precautions require you to treat all clients the same regardless of their age, sex, background, etc. If you are to have contact with any body fluid like urine, blood, etc., you are to treat that fluid as infected and having the potential to transmit disease. You wear clean gloves when any direct exposure is possible and, if the exposure may warrant it, you wear other protective equipment like goggles, gown, mask, etc. You will receive valuable classes and information at your school regarding the transmission of disease and how to protect yourself and others from its snare.

Careful and frequent hand washing is the most important manner of protecting yourself and others from the spread of disease. And don't forget your own self-care as a protective measure. All of the rules that your parents taught you about eating good foods, getting enough rest, taking vitamins, and the benefits of exercise are vital in maintaining your health and to prevent illness. Remember, you are in a marathon that you want to finish, so take the precautions that will allow you to make it the whole way to the finish line of a career in nursing.

TO TOUCH A STRANGER

How often in the past week have you had physical contact with a complete stranger? Chances are that those occasions have been rare, and the few you can recall have been incidental. Perhaps it was the quick clasp of hands that comes with an introduction; the brief brush of moving through a crowd; the momentary meeting of fingertips as you receive your change from the cashier. Throughout our lives we unconsciously adhere to the social norms that limit our physical contact with strangers. That is why a nursing education at the clinical site will entail a psychological adjustment on your part that permits you to touch a stranger. And the touch may or may not be pleasant.

Let's address the unpleasant part first. As a nurse, expect to bathe patients who cannot control their urine or bowels. Expect to collect samples of body fluids and excretion to send to the lab for culture and examination. Expect to change purulent and foul-smelling dressings on patients' wounds. Student nurses often say, "I can do a lot, but I cannot stand looking at sputum." Another may say, "I can do a lot, but I can't stand cleaning up people after they vomit because I will probably vomit, too." These reactions are not unusual at all. Many seasoned nurses still gag at certain smells. When that happens, they know to leave the room, take a few breaths, and then return to the room to care for the patient. No one enjoys the experience, but it has to be done. Unpleasant though these situations may be, they actually represent only a small part of the multidimensional role of the nurse. One of the indirect benefits of "getting your hands dirty" (with gloves, of course!) is that you establish your credibility as care giver. By plunging into doing what needs to be done at that moment to ensure your patient's comfort and, hopefully, recovery, you pass a personal test the result of which does not go unnoticed by those around you. You will earn the often unspoken respect of your nursing colleagues, and that of the aides and techs who may ultimately see you as a role model as you soothe your patients through comfort measures. The high regard that aides and techs have for you can pay rich dividends in the form of their vital cooperation in caring for your patients.

Ironically, touching a stranger can be at the same time a personally fulfilling experience. It can be the most rewarding part of your job as a nurse. A professional nurse's job is quite hectic, as divergent needs jockey for position on your mental to-do list. The man down the hall who must go to surgery now; the woman who is complaining of chest pain; the family that is angry with the care being provided—all this will be swirling in your head at the same time. That is why when time allows, spending a few minutes with the curtain closed around your patient, quietly listening to her respiration, and massaging her back with skin care lotion can be the most rewarding experience of your day. The intimacy that you share with these strangers is unsurpassed in any other field. It is the very soul of nursing. You hold the hand of your patients as they discuss their fears the night before major surgery. You console them immediately after they learn that their cancer is terminal. You cradle your patient's new son or daughter, only a few hours old. You reach out for the bereaved son or daughter as you both gaze upon the father who has just breathed his last.

In these instances and a thousand more, your willingness to touch a stranger will allow you the measure of personal satisfaction that can come only from knowing that you have truly helped another human being.

FAST FACTS in a NUTSHELL

- Finding mentors among the clinical staff will accelerate your professional development.
- The use of Standard Precautions to avoid disease and washing your hands is not only a requirement of the facility, but it is common sense as well.
- Get accustomed to physical contact with strangers because that will become an integral part of your nursing practice.

10

Patients as People

INTRODUCTION

As you acquire the nursing skills needed to effectively deal with your client in the clinical setting, remember one thing: The individual you are approaching in the hospital bed was a person long before he was a patient. The constant reference to "the patient" or "the client" in your nursing program could lead you to believe that this population is an unremarkable, homogeneous group. That is not even remotely the case. As you enter the clinical area, expect each patient to be unique just as you would expect each new person you encounter to be unique.

In this chapter, you will learn:

1. It can be the worst of times for your patients.
2. Each patient is unique.
3. Prudence in revealing your own story.

IT CAN BE THE WORST OF TIMES

Imagine this. A 52-year-old woman had a stroke and can move her extremities only to a minimal degree. She cannot speak but understands everything that is occurring around her.

She is clearly afraid. Only last week, she had given a well-received presentation to the corporate board of directors, and the board members were inclined to endorse her proposal. She and her team had then celebrated her great accomplishment at a French restaurant in the city. You are her student nurse and must do a complete head-to-toe assessment and give a complete bed bath. Getting out of bed with your assistance will be your patient's major accomplishment this week.

You will be present at some of the most difficult times that humans can face. Think for a minute about this woman: How would you feel in her situation? She has experienced a catastrophic health event causing everything in her world to change overnight. You will be intimately involved with her at the most challenging time of her life. You may feel uncomfortable and perhaps even ill-prepared to assess, bathe, and get her out of bed. But you must, and the reason is simple. Your patient is depending upon you. You cannot roll back the clock and change the course of events that has led to the patient being placed in this hospital bed. In fact, there is only one thing that you can do, and that is to give your patient the best care possible.

Understand that your patients may not be at their best, and try not to take their occasional rebuffs personally. They are often in some discomfort or affected by the medication they are taking. Recently, a very earnest senior student nurse prepared to care for her client and entered the room after knocking on the door. The response on the other end was, "GET OUT, I AM ON A PRIVATE PHONE CALL."

Her instructor explained that while such rude treatment may feel personal, it generally is not. Experience will help you to distinguish between these lapses in manners and more abusive behavior, which, although rare, should be addressed professionally and assertively with the assistance of your instructor.

EACH PATIENT IS UNIQUE

One day you will provide personal care to a man like Mr. Smith, who is 92 years old and has dementia. You will fully bathe him, clean his mouth, turn him in his bed to prevent sores, and assist him in getting out of bed when he needs to. The identity of this individual transcends that of patient. He is someone's father and another's grandfather. He is a widower who was loved by a devoted wife for many years. And this same Mr. Smith, feeble now and creased with wrinkles, was once the object of great affection among his many brothers and sisters as he smiled and held his toy on his mother's lap. He is a patient, but he was and is a person first.

The following is an excerpt from the nursing journal of then-senior nursing student Laura Giambattista of West Chester University, which appeared in the online edition of *Advance for Nurses* (January 27, 2010). It exquisitely captures the unique person who happens to carry the label of hospital patient:

Lost and Confused

Mr. W, a weak, confused 88-year-old man, was my med/surg patient. He looked at the TV screen with frustration. "Is she talking to me? What is she trying to say? Who is she?"

On the screen Martha Stewart was making turkey balls, laughing and giggling with guests, as Mr. W scowled at her, thinking she was laughing at him. We turned the TV off. Mr. W's confusion and frustration were agonizing. Nurses encouraged him to relax. How could he? He didn't know anyone around him, where he was, why he was there or what time it was. White walls, a wet diaper and a weak body—this is what he felt and saw.

(continued)

(*continued*)

He couldn't sort this sensory input, a jumbled mess of feelings in his body and brain translated into bewilderment and anxiety. He could not lift his weak legs off the bed, such skinny legs; I can barely see muscle.

He was frail, fragile, and distraught. But at one time he was a brawny young man. He fought in WW II at the Battle of the Bulge. Those weak legs were once strong, carrying him through a war; they kept him moving in the Ardennes in one of the worst, coldest battles of that war, where temperatures dipped well below freezing and men froze to death. Those weak legs were once strong, helping Mr. W pick up and run around with his four children. Those weak legs were once strong, walking his two daughters down the aisle and dancing with his long-time wife.

I internalize these thoughts, look at this patient right now and imagine him before I ever knew him. This is a life well lived, who deserves empathy, respect, and compassion. He was most likely independent, lucid and strapping his entire life, and now he lies on the bed, scared, confused, and delicate. That agitation and anxiousness do not seem so baffling anymore, because if I were him, I would feel the same way. The nursing role is beginning to morph into a personal creation for me. The template of what encompasses the role was provided a couple of years ago in school and I think I have added to that skeleton of an explanation through encounters with patients like Mr. W.

Everyone has their own ideas about what the nursing role should emphasize. For me, it is empathy. Empathy is the glue that holds it all together, the muscle to that emaciated "nursing role" skeleton. Empathy doesn't take

(*continued*)

(*continued*)

long; it is not an involved thinking process and it won't add extra mindless work to the day. Empathy is a feeling, an ability to see beyond one's self and the capacity to experience the plight of a patient. Empathy is stopping one's shuffled pace and maybe holding Mr. W's shaking hand, feeling the fear of utter isolation with him, because fear is not so big when you have someone else.

Nursing is an art, and I feel I finally have a canvas, a paintbrush and a magnifying glass to inspect my work. I continue to learn through every patient I come across, and learn even more through introspective thought after the conversations, dissecting the interactions. I will only stop doing this when I have seen it all from every angle and am completely satisfied with my knowledge and ability. This, of course, will never happen, and so I have begun a journey of lifelong learning.

From Giambattista, L. (2010), *Advance for Nurses*, online January 27, 2010.

Laura's poignant reflection beautifully illustrates the fact that "patients are unique." The optimal approach to their care will always recognize that.

PRUDENCE IN REVEALING YOUR OWN STORY

What do you do when the story of your patient is very similar to one that affects you personally? It may be the mother who has just had her third miscarriage; the daughter with abdominal pain who just lost her mother; or the college freshman who is hospitalized for alcohol intoxication. One of these stories sounds very similar to one of yours—or maybe your best friend's story. Do you tell the patient this information to join with him or her to help alleviate their sadness, frustration, embarrassment, or anger? Yes, you may *and* no, you may not!

Sharing personal information with patients can be helpful and may be reasonable if, and only if, the intention of the sharing is to assist the client during his or her difficult life situation. What does that really mean? How can you differentiate when your sharing is for your benefit or for the patient's? Take a moment or two before you share your personal story and reflect on the real reason you feel compelled to tell the patient something personal about yourself. Are you obsessing about your own story and just looking for an opportunity to tell someone? Could it be that this patient is so nice and welcoming and you feel so comfortable with her, and you need to tell someone?

Your professional responsibility as a nurse is to render nursing care that will benefit and help the patient achieve his or her goals while in your care. The patient is not there to listen to your story. Here are some examples that may assist you in deciding when it is appropriate to share personal information about yourself and when it is not:

Situation 1: Joe's Story

Nurse Joe's father is currently in a center city neuro ICU after sustaining a stroke. Joe has been at his father's bedside for the past 5 days and now, while his father is somewhat stabilized, has returned to work since he is out of benefit time.

Joe is caring for an 89-year-old woman who has dementia and now is hospitalized with pneumonia. This woman is not improving and the medical team is discussing her need for a ventilator. The patient does not have a living will or advance directive. Her two daughters are on the unit and discussing what their next actions need to be for their mother. Joe feels strongly that the patient should be placed on a ventilator for a brief time to see if her pneumonia will heal. He feels that it would be wrong to just let this woman decompensate on his unit and not be transferred to ICU. He is entering the patient's room to state his opinion to the two daughters when his "little voice" stops him. He heeds that voice, and he asks another nurse to cover for him and takes a 10-minute break from the unit. He just pauses and reflects on what is motivating him to talk to the two daughters. During this brief pause, he realizes that he is being influenced by his own family situation. His father is 82 and has been on a ventilator for 6 days now. His father did not have a living will and the family really was not asked about the ventilator during this acute crisis. He realizes that he is too close to this scenario and would unduly influence his patient's daughters with his own story. Since giving his perspective would not be solely for the benefit of the patient, he decides not to voice his opinion to the daughters.

Situation 2: Brianna's Story

Brianna is working on a cardiac unit. She is caring for a woman who may need heart surgery. This woman's condition is unstable and the hospital is a small community hospital that performs about 15 cardiac surgeries per year. Brianna has cared for this woman and has gotten to know her family well. The family asks her one evening what she would do about having the surgery at this facility if the patient were her own mother. What should Brianna say? She also decided to take a few minutes of reflection before she answers the family's questions. As a hospital employee, she would not criticize her facility, and she thinks it is a very good one for simple acute health care conditions. She also believes that to increase the chances for a successful outcome, the patient needs to be in a larger facility with more experience in cardiac surgery.

After gathering her thoughts, she told the family that she believes in obtaining second opinions for all recommended procedures and surgeries. By simply stating this one fact, she does not criticize her own hospital and allows the client and her family to pursue their own course. Brianna has been able to stay true to her own beliefs without compromising her professional responsibility.

There is a boundary between you and your clients. You are a professional who is there solely for the patient's welfare and benefit. Expect patients to ask for your opinion, as nurses are often the most trusted of all professionals. Follow the simple rule of sharing only personal information that would benefit the patient. Do not give the patient your telephone number or any other identifying personal information. It is not professional, and depending upon the patient it may not even be safe. You can share generalizations like, "I live near school," but not the address of your home. If a patient becomes too familiar, insists on having your telephone number, and makes statements like, "You are the only person that I can talk to about this"—beware! Cultivating a personal relationship from a professional one is not appropriate, and you would be in jeopardy if you pursued this course. As a student, always speak to your nursing instructor about any situation in which you feel uncomfortable or if the patient or family is persistent in asking for personal information about you.

FAST FACTS in a NUTSHELL

- You are often seeing patients at the very worst times in their lives. Don't take occasional rebuffs personally.
- Each patient that every nurse cares for is someone's treasured family member or dear friend. Treat each patient with the empathy that you would want your own loved ones treated with.
- Exercise caution in revealing personal information to patients.

In Student Nurses' Own Words . . .

"Keep a positive attitude and take the initiative to learn (it took me a while to get this one . . .). Don't procrastinate with assignments. Understand that they help you formulate your thought process and allow the instructor to show you better ways to care for your clients. Clients are real people, just like myself."

"Rely on your fellow students. We helped each other and learned from each other. Take advantage of experience by asking questions of your instructor and the nurses who work at the clinical site. Even the bad ones can teach you how not to communicate! The reality of the nursing world is high patient-to-nurse ratios. I was not prepared for how physical nursing really is."

"Clinical was difficult for me, and it was helpful to remind myself that it was a phase I just needed to get through to get to where I want in my career. Electronic devices are useful, but not necessary. Your med book is all you need in clinical. If you are careful with your medication administration, you will be fine."

"I loved every rotation. Go in expecting to have fun and you will learn a lot."

"Clinical is not as stressful as everyone thinks. You do not need to know all of the information—just know where to find it."

"Be sure to prepare for clinical by knowing basics like lab values, assessments, and important procedures. Get a PDA for meds. Use your patho book a lot for research. Do not feel out of place at the clinical site—you belong there."

"Documentation is a huge part of nursing. Work with others in a positive and respectful manner. You have to help each other."

"Keep your eye out for learning opportunities. Don't wait for people to ask you to do things."

"Include a couple of professional articles in your journal about topics relating to clinical. The professors will be impressed that you went the extra mile. Take a deep breath and don't be scared. You are just a student, and it is hard to make mistakes if you ask for help when you need it."

"Be clear on what the instructor's expectations of you are."

"Use the course syllabus to make sure you understand what the expectations of you are in clinical. Having an evaluation midway through the clinical rotation is useful in identifying your strengths and weaknesses."

"Establish a rapport with your clinical instructor. Know what they are looking for and talk to students who have had them before for their impressions. Have a handy resource for drug names and medical terms. I prefer a book but others like electronics. Practice your clinical skills in the school's lab."

"Be extremely nice to your clinical instructor and let them see that you are trying to learn. Rather than having a point

system for grades, your grade is based on what the clinical instructor thinks you deserve."

"Don't be afraid to speak up. Sometimes you will catch things before the nurse does. Work with your fellow students. Teach them what you know and learn from them when you are not sure how to do something. Most patients like having nursing students because they get extra attention, so don't be scared of them."

If I could do it over again, I would get an electronic device for drug guides."

"Be sure to get at least eight hours of sleep the night before. Don't hide from your instructor. Utilize her by asking questions."

"My first day was not what I expected. I was timid and nervous. But as the weeks went on I became more confident in interacting with patients and practicing assessment skills."

"I still double-think myself with what procedures to accomplish and when because I get nervous being thrown into a situation. However, it was a great experience. It was interesting to see how the facility needs each person to work together to give effective and quality care to each patient."

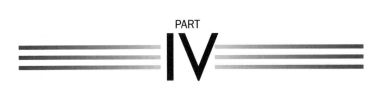

PART

IV

Success at Home

Working, Family, and Crises That Won't Wait

INTRODUCTION

Dorothy Gale had it easy. When the twister blew through her small Kansas town, she was caught up in its vortex and deposited in an unfamiliar place inhabited by unfamiliar people. As a nursing student, can you relate to that dilemma? One advantage Dorothy had in acclimating to her new surroundings was that she could put her former life on hold. While she may occasionally fret for Auntie Em, the fact is that Dorothy could focus pretty much exclusively on following the yellow brick road to her destination. You as a nursing student are not so lucky. Your years in nursing school will likely be complicated by the need to pay for the education you are receiving and dealing with problems that arise within and outside of the family.

In this chapter, you will learn:

1. The do's and don'ts of working while studying.
2. Adjusting family expectations.
3. Coping with crises that won't wait.

THE DO'S AND DON'TS OF WORKING WHILE STUDYING

Economic times are tough! Parents are more concerned than ever that the field of study chosen as their children's college major will be one in which they will be able to procure a job. Adding to this anxiety is the cost of education itself. College tuitions have never been higher than they are right now. The pressure is on students to finish their college degree in four years, not the five- or six-year span that has become increasingly the norm. It is not just a parental concern, as many nursing school students foot the bill for their education on their own. A prime example is seen in the plight of second-degree students who have mortgages, taxes, utility bills, and perhaps their own children's tuition to contend with.

So what will be your decision about working while in nursing school? Prior chapters have clearly described how difficult a major nursing is and how much time you will need to devote to your studies. While you will ideally not need to work over the course of your education, but financial realities may dictate otherwise. Holding a job while matriculating as a nursing student can be done if the work/study balance is managed wisely or if there is a support system in place to cook your meals, wash your clothes, do your food shopping, etc. Also acknowledge that the ability to juggle a job and your coursework becomes even more complex if you also have dependent children. Remember that nursing school requires many more hours beyond those spent in the classroom or at the clinical site. Both classroom and clinical courses require much preparation.

The best advice to hear when determining your ability to live the double life as a worker and student is to use common sense. One student worked as a bartender until 2:00 a.m. of the same morning in which she was scheduled to appear at the clinical site a mere five hours later. For all of her ambition, she did not manage her student life well and it was evident in her clinical performance.

Conversely, working on weekends or some evenings when classes finish at 10:00 a.m. or 12:00 noon is reasonable. The best advice of all is to get a job as a nursing aide or nurse extern and thereby become exposed to the hospital or nursing home setting before you enter it as a nursing student. The experience that you will acquire in that type of job will increase your confidence level and enhance your performance when you begin to interact with patients and staff as a student nurse. Perhaps most important, this additional dimension of working in a health care facility can one day make you a more attractive candidate for a nursing position once you have obtained your license.

The maximum that most nursing students can work and still be healthy and sane is about 20 hours a week, give or take. While on semester breaks and summers, many students work full time to save money for the school semesters when their course load will demand that they work fewer hours. Occasionally, there are students who, for whatever reason, try to keep a full-time job while at the same time studying to become a nurse. It is usually not a successful outcome, and it often jeopardizes both their success in school and their health.

ADJUSTING FAMILY EXPECTATIONS

One of the best pieces of advice that one can give any intrepid soul who steps out onto the road leading to a nursing career is to have a long and honest conversation with your friends and loved ones before you begin your first semester. Often the profile of the person who enters nursing school is that of the "caretaker." They are the ones who organize the family get-togethers, visit with aging parents and take them to their appointments, help their neighbors with babysitting, listen to friends about their many problems, and so on. Perhaps it is the caretaker in you that has attracted you to the nursing profession to begin with.

Laudable though the efforts of the caretaker may be, your decision to enter nursing school will necessitate some degree of modification in your caretaker role. All of the people who are accustomed to relying on you should be forewarned of the limits of your availability. To emphasize your point, consider a family meeting. Bring a copy of the curriculum and nursing handbook. They should see with their own eyes that you will need to maintain a B average to continue in the program. They need to see that every weekend you will be at a clinical site from 7:00 a.m. to 7:00 p.m. Yes, you may have always been a good student, but you never were a nursing student before. As a student at a clinical site for two days a week, you will be expected to prepare and do lengthy homework assignments, care plans, and journals relating to your clinical experiences. You will have exams weekly or every other week that cover seven chapters of intensely detailed information and have little advice on what specifically you will be tested on. Your family and friends need to know that you will not be able to organize and cook the dinners to the same extent as before, and there will be times when you yourself will not have time to join the group at a dinner organized and cooked by someone else while you are in the grasp of nursing school.

Thank them for their patience and consideration of your plight. Remind them that the situation is a temporary one, and you will eventually return as a person who, with their support, has achieved a challenging and rewarding personal goal.

COPING WITH CRISES THAT WON'T WAIT

Mary had always thought about becoming a nurse. In college, her grades were not high enough to transfer into nursing from communications, so she completed her degree and worked for four years as a communications director for a small skilled nursing home near her home. She enjoyed her work and loved the residents but the little voice inside her kept saying, "What about nursing?" She would wistfully observe the nursing staff in her facility rendering care to the residents and imagine herself in this role. When her mother suddenly became sick and passed away after a massive heart attack, Mary could no longer accept placing her heart's desire to become a nurse on hold. She had directly witnessed the skill and kindness that the nursing staff rendered to her mother and, with the support of her family, began traversing the path to nursing.

Her first semester went well. She left her full-time job and worked part-time as a receptionist. Despite getting only six hours of sleep each night rather than her customary eight hours, she was energized by the actualization of her dream of becoming a nursing student. During her second semester, the floor dropped from under her when her four-year-old child developed asthma. It descended suddenly in the middle of the night and she and her husband had to rush him to the emergency room. She missed two class and clinical days, and the director of the program notified her that she may need to take a leave from the program since she had already missed more time than permitted due to the accelerated nature of the program. What a crisis! What should she do? She had waited for all of this time and finally had an opportunity to fulfill her life's dream but the health of her child was at stake. The pediatrician had cautioned the parents that any added stress to the four-year-old child may precipitate more episodes of asthmatic attacks. Hiding her stress would not be easy. Mary worked every weekend at the skilled nursing facility and was a full-time nursing student, wife, mother of two, and sole child of her widower father.

What would you suggest for Mary? This scenario is not too far from reality. Just because you have decided to enter nursing school and to accept its demanding price, the rest of your life does not go on automatic pilot. Children get ill. Parents become dependent. Work responsibilities continue and life partners will expect you to continue to meet their needs. The goal is to balance all of these needs if indeed that is possible. Doing so takes creative thinking and careful planning.

Mary hired a babysitter who lived two doors down from her home, a young college student who was looking for work. Mary arranged it so that the college student, Kristen, came every other day and took her children to the park, performed light housekeeping duties in the home, and prepared dinner on those days for the family. While it was an expense that Mary and her spouse could not easily afford, they knew that they needed to get this kind of help. Mary also found an agency that would assist her elderly widower father with his appointments, shopping, and companionship. She went to the director of her nursing program and listed all of the above adjustments that she made with her family and offered to make up the clinical time she missed (for which she had to pay extra to cover the nursing instructor's salary).

Mary also adjusted her sights grade-wise. She was satisfied to achieve "Bs" in her nursing courses, realizing that it was not worth the anxiety that would come with the treasured "A." She began talking to one of her professors, who told her that most of her best, most successful, and happy students were the "B" students who had attained some degree of life balance. Throughout it all, Mary found tremendous value in practicing some of the "self-care" skills that are discussed in Chapter 12.

While Mary was able to overcome the obstacles that impeded her educational journey, others may not be as successful. Sometimes personal crises are such that no amount of creative thinking or careful planning can surmount them. In these extreme cases, the best course of action to take in managing an unexpected life crisis is to request an official Leave of Absence. This middle road between struggling along as a student and dropping out of the program entirely is appropriate when the personal crisis can be expected to resolve itself within a reasonable period of time. While getting approval of your request is not a sure thing, it is nonetheless in your interest to go to the director of the nursing program, explain the situation, and explore the ramifications of taking a leave for a semester or even a year. Yes, it may delay your graduation, but in the end you still will have achieved your goal of becoming a nurse despite having to navigate through the turbulent tides of personal crises.

═══════════════════════*FAST FACTS in a NUTSHELL*

- Working while in nursing school takes careful planning to avoid compromising the effectiveness of your education.
- Family members need to be informed up-front that your need to commit to your studies may limit your availability to them.
- Creative thinking can sometimes allow a nursing student to handle personal crises without unduly impacting progress toward graduation.

12

You Are Your Own Patient

INTRODUCTION

Before any commercial airline leaves the ground, the flight attendant stands before the travelers to demonstrate the safety features of the aircraft. When it comes to the oxygen mask, the advice is always the same: Apply your own oxygen mask before assisting others. The logic is simple. You are of little value in assisting another individual if you yourself are depleted. As an aspiring nurse, you will begin to understand that you are your own patient.

In this chapter, you will learn:

1. The need to sleep, eat, and have fun.
2. The value of relaxation, exercise, and meditation.
3. When to seek counseling.

As a student nurse, the first patient you must care for will be yourself.

THE NEED TO SLEEP, EAT, AND HAVE FUN

You can anticipate long days both as a student in the classroom and at a clinical site where you may face a twelve-hour shift. Prepare properly for each day by planning for your consumption of sufficient food and drink. Do not depend on potato chips, candy bars, and other vending machine fare to meet your nutritional needs. School and health care facility cafeterias can be options if they offer a healthy variety and reasonable pricing. Otherwise, don't be reluctant to carry an insulated food bag like you did in grade school (without the latest TV character or action figure). Make yourself a sandwich (peanut butter and jelly is nutritious and cheap) accompanied by fruit, multigrain chips, real juice or milk, and yes, something with caffeine to give you that pick-up you will need in the afternoon. It will be well worth those few extra minutes the night before or the day of clinical to ensure that you will have enough fuel to get you through the day.

When the house, apartment, or dorm room finally gets quiet at 10:00 p.m., it can be a great time to study; that is, assuming you do not have to awaken before 6:00 a.m. for class or clinical. A recent grad and varsity soccer player told her instructor at the end of the clinical day that she went to bed at 2:00 a.m. following a night game at the opponent's field. She needed to awaken by 5:00 a.m. to be at her clinical med-surg site by 6:15 a.m. Although she managed to get through the day without any problem, she admitted that she could not do this on a regular basis. Studies have documented that a minimum amount of sleep, approximately six to seven hours, is necessary for superior cognitive functioning. Please believe that you need superior cognitive functioning! Given the importance of a good night's rest in performing capably the following day, consider these recommendations for sleep hygiene:

- Go to bed and arise the same times each day (even on days off). Your body must know it is getting near to bedtime and begin to release melatonin, which promotes sleep.
- Do not go to bed hungry. Eat cheese, crackers, cereal, milk, a small sandwich, or some other food with protein and a little fat.
- No TV in your room, but if you must, turn it off at least an hour before bedtime.
- Keep the bedroom cool.
- Try not to take daytime naps. If you must, keep them to fifteen or twenty minutes.
- Limit caffeine intake (tea, coffee, soda, energy drinks) from about 4:00 p.m. on. They take up to six hours to completely be cleared from your system.
- Exercise daily even for fifteen minutes. Don't exercise within a few hours of bedtime.
- Practice meditation or listen to soothing music to begin to relax your brain before going to bed.
- If you find your head spinning with "to-do" lists, get out of bed, write down what needs to be accomplished, and give it up to the next day.

Build some time for fun into your schedule and get to know your classmates outside of class. Don't be surprised if some become lifelong friends. In later years, you will look back with them and laugh at the fun you managed to squeeze out of your nursing school days. Go out to a restaurant for dinner or relax with them at a local pub. Not only are you making memories, but the release you temporarily feel from the rigor of the educational demands you share can be a welcome tonic for your beleaguered brain.

When the weekend comes, try to set aside a full day when you do not do any work associated with nursing school. You will be able to return to your work more refreshed if you do. Avoid becoming "burned out" by getting caught in a cycle of working and studying with no time left for "you."

RELAXATION, EXERCISE, AND MEDITATION

The restorative effects of having fun as just described are shared with other more benign pursuits. To achieve the level of relaxation you need in a balanced life, give yourself permission to take a breather when you feel that you need one. Walk in the park, read a fun book, telephone a friend, cook something special, watch a movie, attend your children's soccer games, and so on. At least one former nursing student confessed that her secret source of relaxation is spending time alone working on "paint-by-number" illustrations. Any activity that allows the nursing brain to lie fallow for a few hours pays dividends in sharper cognition once it is time to get back to task. Perhaps the two best ways to relax are exercise and meditation.

Exercise prompts your own natural endorphins (i.e., "feel-good" brain chemicals) to be secreted. A brisk walk three times a week will help keep your weight stable and avoid the "freshman twenty." Working out in the gym three times a week will help keep your muscle tone intact, and walking on a treadmill will turn on the endorphin faucet as well.

Many students lament the fact that they have not gone to the gym in weeks because of all of their school work. This is not productive. Allow yourself to exercise (even in a more limited fashion) at least three times a week during your school days.

To many, meditation conjures the image of a guru sitting on a cushion with hands uplifted while chanting. Actually, meditation can take other forms that fit more easily into Western culture. All have the same goal of sifting out the situational distracters of the moment and the anxiety they convey. One simple method of meditation you can practice is learning to slow your breath. Breathing in through your nose to the count of four and exhaling through your mouth to the count of five for three consecutive times may be enough to lower the stress effect on your body when done several times a day.

Picture this scenario. Your instructor is walking down the hospital hallway to observe you preparing and administering medications to your patient. Your patient happens to be a 65-year-old physician and knows all about her medications. Unfortunately, you have not done this procedure often in your student nursing experience. Your sympathetic nervous system goes into overdrive. You begin to sweat, your breathing speeds up, you feel a little sick to your stomach, and your brain starts to freeze! Should you run, freeze, or fight? Why not take three deep breaths and close your eyes for just a second or two and really concentrate only on your breath? This simple breathing exercise will likely tap into your parasympathetic nervous system, which is designed to calm you down and allow your brain to concentrate in a more efficient way.

Learning simple meditation techniques and practicing them at home, in the supermarket line, or while waiting at the dentist office will allow you to shift more quickly to these techniques during a stressful period as a nursing student. Achieving relaxation through breathing modulation can be particularly effective in alleviating test anxiety. Suppose that you are now taking that all important nursing exam that they say is "really difficult." You feel your body tensing and your sympathetic nervous system starting again. Remember to take those deep breaths. You can take them quietly or with a sigh (go to the bathroom and sigh out loud if you like before an exam).

These techniques have been found helpful in reaching full concentration and optimal brain performance. If you find that helpful, you can go even further. Go online or retrieve an app for your iPhone and actually listen to a brief meditation before a clinical or exam.

WHEN TO SEEK COUNSELING

What is normal versus abnormal stress? When are symptoms of obsessive-compulsive disorder under control and actually useful, and when are they not functional? When do you need to seek counseling or therapy?

We all have idiosyncratic habits and anxieties. In today's world with everyone saying things like "I am so depressed today" or "I am going crazy," how can one differentiate when counseling is really needed? One simple rule to remember is that if a certain habit, feeling, thought, or action (or lack of action) is interfering with your daily life, you should seek assistance. Interference would indicate that the habit, feeling, thought, or action is negatively affecting your interaction with family, friends, and associates at work.

Many schools have a very helpful counseling department where, if needed, you can be seen on the same day of your telephone call. They can screen and assist you in your decision to know if you need to continue in counseling. The counseling departments in most schools have therapists who will see you for several visits. They also have access to referral resources that specialize in your particular need. This service is usually part of your tuition or involves a minimal fee.

If you have a recurring concern that is hampering your success as a nursing student, do not suffer in silence. Talk over your symptoms with a friend or trusted faculty member. Alternately, if your situation is stable but you find a fellow student who is struggling, encourage that student to seek counseling, even going so far as to walk the troubled student to the counseling department if that is acceptable to him or her.

One final note: If you have any thoughts of self-harm or harming someone else, you must immediately seek help from a faculty member or call the school counseling department. In off hours, contact the security office. If it is a fellow student who exhibits the same behavior, follow the same steps. You may be saving a life.

FAST FACTS in a NUTSHELL

- Now more than ever, your health depends on proper sleep and diet.
- Build time into your schedule to relax and have fun.
- Discover counseling resources that are available to you if you need them.

In Student Nurses' Own Words . . .

"There really isn't a balance—it's either all school or not. I spent weekends doing homework, but I did make sure to do one social event each week. Eat a good dinner and keep a regular bedtime. Do homework in a comfortable place—even outside if the weather allows."

"Setting priorities is key, and is a calming force. Although priorities are always shifting between school and family, it was usually possible to keep a balance. School can be very stressful and it is important to have a life outside of all of that stress—something to keep you grounded. My fellow classmates were a good support system. We were all going through that same stuff together and that commonality was a great comfort at times."

"Change your opinion of what is a good grade or you will be disappointed. Get to know the faculty."

"Manage your time and manage the stress of life's difficulties so that they do not affect your concentration with school. Running and going to church helped to decrease my stress. I saved the weekends to socialize and still managed to get my work done. You cannot go out and 'party' like you did in freshman year. Junior and senior years are hard, but you will get it done and be out before you know it."

"It's like walking a tightrope. Sometimes you have balance and sometimes you feel wobbly. But you see the finish and no matter what has happened you will get to the end. Get a job in health care to avoid getting to the end and deciding that nursing is not right for you."

"Make sure you sleep and go out to have fun. Study before exams and go out after."

"Make time for yourself to relax. Keep your family close and involved, because you are going to need people to talk and vent to. Apply for externships in your junior year. Manage your time wisely. Make lists and use a calendar. Plan ahead to get your work done so you can have some free time on the weekend."

"Learn to love the library. Going with friends can even make it a fun/social experience."

"Stay on top of your work. Once you fall behind, it is easy to drown. Try hard and don't get down on yourself when you do not get that 'A.' Nursing school is hard. Don't be surprised if you are jealous of your friends who slack off and party every day of the week while you are working your butt off. It will be worth it in the end."

"Make sure nursing is what you really want because it is a lot of work but worth it in the end."

"If you find a nursing-related job before junior year, it will be easier to find a nursing job after graduation."

"Getting a job as a nurse's aide will give you added confidence in clinical and also be helpful later in getting a job as a nurse."

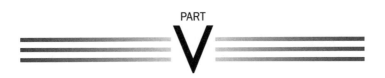

PART

V

Success Following Graduation

Licensure

INTRODUCTION

Remember the euphoria you experienced when you received your driver's license? By demonstrating your ability to safely drive a car, you were given official permission to get behind the wheel and travel in whatever direction you chose. Similarly, after several years of preparation and demonstrating your ability to perform safely in your chosen profession, you will experience that same thrill again with the acquisition of your nursing license.

In this chapter, you will learn:

1. The process of applying for a nursing license.
2. The impact of a criminal past on licensing.
3. About temporary practice permits.

Obtaining a nursing license represents the culmination of your ardent efforts during your years as a nursing student. Your nursing license will finally open doors to a career in nursing.

THE PROCESS OF APPLYING FOR A NURSING LICENSE

A nursing license is obtained from the state board of nursing. Go to your state's Web site and find the tab that relates to licenses. You should find nursing among the professions that require a license, and follow the directions provided. Your application for a nursing license triggers a process that ultimately ensures that the candidate is sufficiently skilled to begin actual practice. Upon receipt of your application and completion of a review of your educational credentials, the state will provide you with instructions regarding registration for the NCLEX® (National Council Licensing Examination). The licensing candidate must pass this qualifying exam before a license will be awarded. Along with the instructions you will receive an "Authorization to Test" letter from the state. This letter is a prerequisite for NCLEX registration. After taking the test, your score will be calculated by the NCLEX administrator and conveyed to the state board of nursing. It is the state board of nursing that will inform you of the NCLEX result. For additional information regarding NCLEX, visit www.ncsbn.org/nclex

The NCLEX is covered more fully in Chapter 14.

THE IMPACT OF A CRIMINAL PAST ON LICENSING

The pursuit of a nursing license offers yet one more proof that crime does not pay. If it does not preclude you from getting a license, it can at least make the process more tenuous. The impact of a past criminal conviction on your acquisition of a nursing license will be a function of two things: (1) the nature of the conviction itself and (2) a particular state's stance on allowing applicants with a criminal past into its nursing ranks.

All states require a criminal background check as part of the licensing process for nurses. How they interpret the results in terms of the applicant's suitability to become a nurse can vary from state to state. Unless a given state has a zero tolerance policy with respect to criminal convictions, each case must be considered individually. Obviously, the less serious misdemeanors (such as shoplifting) will be given different weight than the more serious felonies (such as armed robbery). There may be one conviction on a person's record or there may be several. The conviction may have occurred last month or two decades ago. Some convictions may even have been expunged from a person's record. In any event, it is strongly advisable for any aspiring nurse with a criminal past to clearly understand the state's position on granting licenses to such individuals before investing personal resources in a career that could be out of reach.

ABOUT TEMPORARY PRACTICE PERMITS

In states that make them available, the temporary practice permit allows the graduate nurse to assume job duties *before* successfully completing the NCLEX. The use of temporary practice permits is usually in response to a nursing shortage. In these instances, new grads procure this permit, are hired, and begin their orientation on their new units. While working on the basis of a temporary practice permit, the graduate nurse must operate under the supervision of a licensed registered nurse who is physically on the same unit. At some point the graduate nurse would take and pass the NCLEX within a prescribed timeframe, all the while continuing seamlessly in his or her professional role.

A job market with no nursing shortage diminishes the need for temporary practice permits. Call or visit online area hospitals and find out their policy on new graduate hiring practices.

FAST FACTS in a NUTSHELL

- Nursing licenses are obtained through the State Board of Nursing.
- A criminal background can impede or prevent the acquisition of a nursing license.
- Temporary practice permits may be available in times of nursing shortages to allow graduate nurses to begin work before obtaining a license.

14

NCLEX® (The National Council License Examination)

INTRODUCTION

After a lot of hard work, you have successfully completed your nursing education program. Congratulations on your accomplishment! Ready to go to work? Not so fast! In most if not all jurisdictions there is a standard test that stands between you and your nursing license. The National Council Licensure Examination (NCLEX®) must be passed by the new nursing school graduate before obtaining the coveted nursing license.

In this chapter, you will learn:

1. To begin preparing on day 1.
2. About books, CDs, and online resources.
3. Whether to take a prep class.

Like members of many other professions, such as lawyers, physical therapists, and physicians, nursing program graduates must pass a state licensing exam before they are legally qualified to practice. As a nursing student, you will one day face the NCLEX (National Council Licensure Examination for Registered Nurses)—the nursing board exam of the state in which you intend to be licensed. Even if you were to earn your nursing degree, you cannot practice as a registered nurse unless you pass the nursing board exam!

It does not matter which course of study has been taken—associate, diploma, or baccalaureate; all take the same licensing exam for registered nurses. (There is an exam for licensed practical nurses as well but the state regulations are different from those governing registered nurses.) Knowing the importance of the NCLEX, some prospective nursing students will select a nursing program based on its NCLEX pass rate in comparison to other schools. Go to your state's licensing board Web site; these scores should be readily available.

Not surprisingly, the NCLEX is comprehensive. It is taken at a testing center with questions posed and responded to via a computer. The length of the NCLEX will vary, as an incorrect answer can prompt additional questions to ascertain actual depth of knowledge. Figure on having to answer approximately 100 to 250 questions in the time allotted. At this writing, the cost of the NCLEX is $200 along with administrative fees, which are determined by each individual state.

Getting a little more time on an exam to be able to read the questions thoroughly or being tested in a room alone, which would be distraction free, could make the difference between success or not. Remember that if you were eligible for testing accommodations in your course of study in school, you also are eligible when you take the NCLEX.

BEGIN PREPARING ON DAY 1

A word to the wise: Don't wait until three months before you plan to take the nursing board exam to practice answering the type of questions you are going to encounter. Begin preparing for the board exam right from the start of your nursing studies. The more exposure you have to how the threads of nursing concepts can be woven into questions, the more adept you will be at answering them correctly when acquisition of your license depends on it.

So what exactly is meant by beginning preparation for the NCLEX on day 1? At the end of each chapter of your nursing texts, you should find questions usually described as NCLEX-style questions. Your nursing professor may require you to answer them; they may appear in your nursing exams; or they may not even be mentioned by the teacher of the course. Regardless of the treatment they are given in the classroom, their ultimate importance to you as a learning tool is undiminished.

Preparation for the NCLEX will begin with your initial level 100 or 200 course, which will be called "Fundamentals of Nursing" or something similar. It teaches nursing theories, nursing assessment, basic hygiene principles, and Standard Precautions to be exercised by nurses. This introductory course constitutes the conceptual scaffolding you will need before traveling to clinical sites later in your nursing program. Find and answer the NCLEX questions at the end of the chapter. Alternately, these questions are online, and the textbook publisher gives you a code along with purchase of the textbook. If you rent or use a text online, you should have access to these questions as well. Whatever source is used, it will instruct you where you can find the correct answers, whether provided online or in the back of the textbook.

Recall an important observation from earlier in this book: Most beginning nursing students have difficulty with nursing questions. These questions are different from most other fields of study. They often require you to assimilate the information and then apply it to a certain situation. There will often be at least two answers that appear correct. Your job as you answer all NCLEX-style questions is to study the formatting of the questions and the formatting of the answers and then begin to decipher the pattern of logic for these questions.

The key to success here is practice! The more NCLEX-style questions you tackle, the more familiar you will become with their patterns and subtleties. One nursing professor who is well acquainted with the NCLEX had this to say: "To obtain the most benefit from NCLEX review questions, **the quality of the review is more important than the quantity.**" What did she mean? Here is an illustration. Review the questions with two sources nearby, like *Taber's Cyclopedic Medical Dictionary* and a medications resource. As you read each review question, avoid the temptation to skip over questions containing terms or medications with which you are not familiar. Try to answer them, and then, even if you have answered correctly, look up each term or medication that you do not know. The time invested here in deepening your knowledge base will yield a greater benefit than you would otherwise receive by simply answering additional questions.

Do not get frustrated with your initial test scores. They will likely improve as you move further into your nursing studies. What if they do not? Many nursing programs have developed an academic support course that students can take to buttress their knowledge. This course usually gives tips for success in taking the NCLEX and enumerates different test-taking strategies that may be very helpful in exam success. In fact, there are some nursing schools that mandate academic support for struggling students (e.g., a course grade that is below 77) before allowing them into the next required nursing course.

Just as your success on the NCLEX is important to you, it is also important to your school. Many states have penalties in place if a nursing school's NCLEX pass rate falls below a certain level. The state has the jurisdiction to place that school on probation and mandate certain program changes. Therefore, it is not surprising that nursing schools commonly provide built-in assistance to help ensure your success with NCLEX. They may even require students to take NCLEX-style online exams, which the students must purchase from companies like Evolve or ATI. The resultant test score can be combined with their classroom grades to yield a final grade for the course. You take these exams during your regular class time in conditions that are somewhat similar to what you may find with your state board licensing exam. This includes but is not limited to a specified time interval and bringing nothing into the room except you and a form of identification. The school will provide the computer you will use to take the exam, and it will have a calculator feature for your use. You will not be able to bring your own calculator, smartphone, or any similar device into the exam room. These practice tests are a real bonus for you. Despite your normal anxiety about the grade that you receive, they subject you to experience, in a limited way, the NCLEX exam. If you fare poorly in a particular test topic—pharmacology or pediatrics, for instance—appreciate the forewarning it represents. You have evidence of your need to invest additional study in this area before you take the NCLEX "for real." In fact, your school may require you to take a review course before you can sit for the NCLEX.

During junior and senior year, you will take NCLEX-style exams on specific subject areas. Most schools then have a cumulative-type exam that occurs in the spring of their senior year and is designed to mimic the official NCLEX. It has become standard for many schools to require that you reach a certain score in this "RN exit exam" as a condition of successfully completing the nursing program. For example, the passing score for one school's RN exit exam is 850 and would typically be reflected in the Student Handbook as follows: "Attaining a score of 850 is required on the RN exit exam for the director of the program to sign off on your application to sit for the NCLEX exam."

BOOKS, CDs, AND ONLINE RESOURCES

There are specific books that many students purchase containing a plethora of NCLEX-style questions divided into such pertinent subheadings as Pediatrics, Maternity, Medical-Surgical, Psychiatric, Community, Pharmacology, and Management and Delegation. Like other successful students, you can purchase one of these books after completing each course of study such as medical-surgical and any related clinical component. Alternately, you can download apps that have countless NCLEX-style questions onto your smartphone. Then, when you have time between classes or laundry cycles, or traveling out on the road (as the passenger, not the driver!), you can review these questions at your convenience.

To use these resources to their maximum effectiveness, it is recommended to wait until you actually begin your nursing courses. Some programs do not introduce nursing courses to nursing majors until their spring semester of sophomore year or even into junior year. It could prove frustrating to begin this NCLEX review and preparation while you are busily completing the science prerequisites needed before entering nursing courses.

The students' ability to correctly answer questions posed in the book in the subject area they have just completed allows them to ascertain whether their knowledge base is sufficient or whether it needs reinforcement. Having received an "A" in a given nursing course and another "A" in its clinical component is not necessarily a predictor of NCLEX success. Ultimately, your readiness to take the NCLEX will largely be a product of the level of effort you have given in your own learning process, and the level of expertise of your clinical and classroom instructors in imparting to you what you need to know to function effectively as a nurse. NCLEX text resources have proved to be a very impartial judge in this regard.

Following are some of the resources that nursing students have used in preparing for the NCLEX:

- Mosby's NCLEX Review
- Saunders NCLEX Review
- Hurst Reviews
- HESI Review
- Davis RN Success
- Mosby's Review Flash Cards for the NCLEX-RN
- Springer's NCLEX-RN EXCEL

NCLEX PREP COURSES

In the fall or spring of your senior year, you will be bombarded with different advertisements about NCLEX review courses. A review course should be considered by those who were less than diligent in their NCLEX preparation as they progressed through the nursing program and as a capstone by others who wish to have the essence of their studies distilled into one densely packed week. While potentially valuable to individuals such as these, be sure to read the fine print before signing on. Pay particular attention to the program's policies in the event of subsequent NCLEX failure, and the NCLEX pass/fail rates among those who have taken the course previously.

There are differing styles and types of review courses available to you. One is instructor-led in a classroom setting. This review course is typically five days long and lasts from 9:00 a.m. to 2:00 p.m. Larger vendors have multiple sites offering the onsite option. In addition to personal instruction, these courses give you access to a multitude of online NCLEX-type questions that you can continue to practice. If you do better with personal instruction and its attendant time structure, consider this review course option and be sure to sign up early to avoid being closed out as enrollment can be limited. On the other hand, suppose you live in a more remote area or have commitments such as small children to care for. The opportunity to attend a classroom review course is necessarily limited for you. In that case, an online review course may be a better fit.

In either mode, courses generally come with guarantees. These guarantees might state that if you take the NCLEX within six months of graduation and completion of the review course but do not pass the exam, you will receive your money back minus an administration fee. They also may offer a remediation course or even a tutor at no additional cost if you prefer this option. The average cost for either type of review course can range from $350 to $500 depending on the area of the country where you live.

Solicit input from prior graduates from your school regarding the effectiveness of these review courses and listen to their impression about the wisdom of taking these courses. Many students say, "I am taking it because I do not want to regret not taking it." Many nursing school graduates discuss this decision with their fellow graduates and take a course together somewhere. The support of a group that you know and the opportunity of studying together are benefits that have been cited by some students in their NCLEX preparation.

FAST FACTS in a NUTSHELL

- The NCLEX is a standard examination that the nursing graduate must pass in order to acquire a license to practice.
- You can commence with preparation for the NCLEX as soon as your nursing studies begin.
- Books, CDs, and review courses are available to nursing students who want to reinforce their personal knowledge base prior to taking the NCLEX.

15

The Basics of
Job Hunting in Nursing

INTRODUCTION

In nursing, as in other professions, there are two categories of job seekers. Category 1 consists of those lucky few who have a job waiting for them after they graduate. Category 2 is comprised of everyone else. If you are fortunate enough to belong to Category 1, feel free to skip the next two chapters. Category 2 job seekers should read on to get your job search off to a productive start.

In this chapter, you will learn:

1. To plan ahead.
2. How your school can contribute.
3. About externs, interns, and mentors.
4. Sources of job opportunities.

Jobs are usually not obtained by accident. More often, they are the end product of a strategy comprised of various moving parts—figurative gears that interlock and work together to propel forward the process of job hunting. Following are some of the basic moving parts that should be built into a graduate nurse's job-hunting strategy.

PLAN AHEAD

No one can foretell the future with complete accuracy, so planning ahead in formulating a job-hunting strategy is by no means foolproof. Still, a little awareness on your part as to what employers find attractive in an applicant can help.

Consider joining an extracurricular activity. A recent nursing school graduate said, "I wish I had been more involved with on-campus activities such as a nursing club. All of the job applications asked if you were involved in any student organizations. I put 'no' to that question and then had to skip the four or five following questions that then did not pertain to me. If you are involved in on-campus activities or volunteering or something, they ask a bunch of questions about it and you really get to make yourself look good in that section of the application."

Network at each clinical site by talking to each nurse with whom you work. Each person whom you meet during your travels throughout your nursing program may be a potential lead to a job. They were once in your shoes and can be excellent sources of information. Ask them what they did after graduation. What do they like about nursing and what do they not like? Ask them if they would recommend this facility as a place to work. Do they know if there will be any job openings? Could you ever come back and shadow them for a day? The more you familiarize yourself with the "world of nursing" by speaking with the nurses who are active in the field, the better will be your job-hunting prospects.

Find a mentor—an individual whose sage advice will keep you on course as a budding professional. To learn and experience the real spirit of nursing, a mentor can be your key. The mentor is a nurse who also happens to be your neighbor, cousin, faculty member, fellow employee, sibling, or even your parent. They will bestow upon you nuggets of wisdom that help guide you along your career path. Keep your eyes peeled for that person whom you can trust with personal insecurities such as, "I don't even know what to say to a patient." The more time and trust that you establish with your mentor, the more effective may be your job searching and ultimate selection.

EXTERNS, INTERNS, AIDES, AND TECHS

One of the most helpful job-hunting strategies is to choose a health care facility that interests you as a future employer and get in the door now as a nurse extern (also known as a nurse intern), a nurse's aide, or a patient care tech.

Many of today's nurses reached their professional destination by traveling this very route while still in nursing school. Yes, the delicate balance of working while in nursing school has already been established, but the dividends that you will reap by working in the health care field as a student may be priceless.

Generally speaking, a nurse extern is a student nurse who works in an acute care hospital, be it a community hospital or larger teaching facility. Often you are not eligible to apply for this titled position until you complete some of your school's clinical rotations. Many facilities specifically require a medical-surgical clinical rotation before they consider you eligible to be a nurse extern. The extern position is one for which the facility will pay you and train you to perform tasks like taking blood, performing certain aspects of patient care, and other nursing responsibilities. In return, you commit to working during semester breaks and a minimum of a few shifts each month during your school year. Extern positions represent the proverbial "win-win" proposition. They serve to acclimate the student to the real nursing world, while at the same time allowing the manager and staff to observe the nursing student in action. If they like what they see, it is not unusual for the unit manager to suggest that the student apply for a registered nursing position upon graduation. In recent years, this seems to be the most reliable way for nursing graduates to obtain a nursing job upon graduation.

Most of the foregoing information on externship is applicable for nurse's aide and patient care tech positions as well. As the term suggests, the nurse's aide assists the nurse in the completion of tasks relating to patient hygiene and personal care. Health care facilities will usually demand certification (i.e., certified nurse assistant [CNA] certification). Skilled nursing homes employ many nurse's aides.

The patient care tech position requires somewhat more training and involves more responsibility, as they may be asked to draw blood, administer electrocardiograms, and perform other patient care activities.

Unlike externships, neither of these positions has to be filled by a nursing student. Even so, functioning as a nurse's aide or a nursing tech can be valuable to your job prospects as a registered nurse. The nursing staff's awareness of your student nurse status will often prompt them to offer you more opportunities to learn. Here again, the unit manager's personal observance of your punctuality, work ethic, and treatment of the patients can lead ultimately to a promotion to a professional nurse position. Meanwhile, you will be observing the staff and facility to determine if this is a place at which you would like to work.

HOW YOUR SCHOOL CAN CONTRIBUTE

Every school will have a career development center and staff who are there to assist you in your job procurement efforts. They serve all students and often have specific staff members who possess more expertise in individual majors and professional occupations. These essential career counselors often have professional ties to outside employers, which is useful in marketing their school's graduates.

Examples of services offered by a career development center would be the following:

Resume workshops: Assistance in developing a resume that creates a picture of you and opens doors to interviews. You can refine an existing resume or develop one at the workshop.

Drop-in hours: Career center staff members will meet with you to resolve questions and offer guidance.

Resume sharing days: Employers are invited to campus and will provide tips and feedback on your resume.

Mock interviews: Develops poise and skill in answering a myriad of questions through practice.

On-campus interview days: Recruiters will be invited to your school and will bring their own marketing techniques. You can bring hard copies of your resume to these events and distribute them to recruiters.

Job postings: Based on the hard work of the Career Development staff, companies, hospitals, schools, and other job advertisers may be listed on the internal career development web site.

As wonderful as the career development center may be, don't forget your teachers as you cast your net for job advice. You have in your nursing faculty a treasure trove of wisdom, connections, and guidance that are yours for the asking. Make connections with the faculty whom you will encounter throughout your education. If a particular faculty member seems to hold more of a personal connection for you, concentrate on that individual's input regarding job options. They can often open doors by pointing you toward a particular person or field in nursing.

SOURCES OF JOB OPPORTUNITIES

Where will the nursing job opportunities be in the future? That is a current debate in the health care world. Some experts expect a large future need in acute care hospitals, especially critical care units. They are predicting that the 70 million baby boomers who are now in their 60s or fast approaching that milestone will be suffering with heart attacks, diabetes, hypertension, and other maladies warranting acute care. Other health care experts are predicting that the opposite will occur—there will be a move away from hospitals in favor of community-based health care settings such as nursing homes, long-term care, home health, and physicians' offices (Stokowski, 2011). Regardless of its locus, there is one thing that everyone can agree on. The need for health care will grow.

Many facilities, especially hospitals, are requiring a BSN degree to be eligible to apply, with a minimum grade point average hovering around 2.8 with a plus or minus factor based on geography. Most will consider your application even if you are currently working at a different facility as long as you have been working about six months or less. If you are a diploma or associate degree nurse, many residency programs will consider your application if you are currently enrolled in an RN-to-BSN program with an anticipated graduation date within a year.

You may want to seek out a facility with a residency program. The advantage here is that often these facilities have "magnet status." Magnet status means that the hospital has been recognized for its excellence and has certain features like shared governance and a clinical ladder for its nurses.

These facilities tend to be more nurse-friendly and are being viewed by the public and nursing worlds as positive places to be treated and employed.

You can begin to probe sources of job opportunities in your junior year by looking at hospital, skilled nursing facility, and home care agency Web sites in search of part-time work. Getting a part-time job in these settings will expose you to nursing in a way that is simply not possible through part-time work in offices, restaurants, supermarkets, and the like.

The majority of new nursing school grads usually obtain their first employment in acute care hospital facilities. That is where the greatest need generally lies. However, if your locale has limited acute care nursing hospital opportunities, consider a skilled nursing home as a place of part-time employment. Many of these facilities take patients following their release from the hospital in order to provide further acute nursing care before the patients' discharge to home. The nurses in skilled nursing facilities tend to become like family to their residents. The speed of turnover is not as fast as in the hospital setting and this gives nurses more of an opportunity to really know their residents. Your assessment and nursing skills will get more finely tuned and improve in these facilities, for often you are the one charged with assessing the resident's need for more intensive care and determining when the physician or other primary care provider needs to be summoned.

More and more hospitals have a residency program for new graduate nurses. They are paid and oriented, unlike years back when new nurses were "thrown in to sink or swim" in their first jobs. To their credit, nursing leaders have come to realize that new grads need transitional assistance upon graduation to learn how to safely care for today's acute patients. This is usually a year-long program that guides you through mentorship, routine support groups and in-services, and other professional opportunities. Nursing

management wants you to stay and be happy after your orientation. Look online early in your nursing career and find
the local hospitals that have residency programs upon graduation for their new nurses. More will be said about nurse
residency programs in Chapter 16.

═══════════════════════════*FAST FACTS in a NUTSHELL*

- An organized approach to finding a job is important.
  Develop a strategy and follow it.
- Your nursing school offers valuable resources in obtaining
  a job following graduation.
- Working part time (even as a student) as a nurse extern,
  aide, or tech can be invaluable in introducing yourself
  to your employer as a potential nurse.

16

The Fine Points of Job Hunting in Nursing

INTRODUCTION

You have completed the marathon. The starting line was your acceptance to nursing school. The finish line is your acquisition of your nursing license. And yet you are still running—this time toward a job. But look around. Others are continuing to run with you toward the same job. Let's separate you from the pack.

In this chapter, you will learn:

1. The crucial value of letters of reference.
2. How to use your network.
3. About interviewing.
4. Persistent (not pesty) follow-up.

The search for a job is ultimately about a professional relationship initiated by one human being and responded to (positively or negatively) by another. As such, a truly effective job search recognizes and gives appropriate weight to this human dimension in differentiating yourself from others like you.

THE CRUCIAL VALUE OF LETTERS OF REFERENCE

Today, more than ever before, letters of reference are an integral part of your job search. Gone are the days when your nursing instructor may just write a form letter of reference, merely changing the name of the designee from letter to letter. Today's nurse recruiters want to know *exactly* who you are. At a recent health system luncheon held for affiliated schools of nursing, the director of the nurse residency program made this statement, "We look and read each application's letters of reference, and are very disappointed when we note that the same letter was used for several applicants by the same nursing faculty member."

As a student, you choose which faculty members will write your letters of reference. In making your request, remember that your nursing faculty members are busy and not always available to comply with your request at short notice. Approach the faculty members in person (preferably) or email and inquire if they would be available to write you a letter of reference. Give them as much forewarning as possible. A minimum of seven to ten days should suffice for most nursing faculty. Be respectful in making your request because faculty members are not required to write reference letters. Below is a sample request from a recent nursing graduate:

Hello XXXX,

Thank you so much for a great rotation on 3C. I cannot think of one negative thing about the rotation (even waking up so early was not so bad by the end). I was

(*continued*)

(continued)

wondering if you would be kind enough to write two letters of recommendation for me, as I plan to apply to both the XXX and XXX health systems this month. I would really appreciate you doing this for me. Please let me know if you are able to write these. My home address would be the best way for me to receive them.

Thank you for your time and for a wonderful clinical rotation!

NAME

ADDRESS

PHONE

Those faculty members who do honor requests for reference letters (which are the large majority) are not necessarily alike in their style of reacting to your need. Some faculty members first require that you fill out a form before they honor your request. Others will have you schedule a follow-up meeting to discuss the content of the letter.

Many students request the letter of reference immediately after they have completed their coursework with the specific instructor. You can choose a classroom faculty member to write your letter, if that is your preference, although many acute care facilities prefer letters of reference from your clinical nursing instructors. The recruiters and nursing management want to hear what your performance is like in the real world of nursing. How did the student react when he had a very challenging patient or family member to contend with? Did the student help and assist the staff and peers while on the unit? Employers are looking for both good grades and personality qualities like poise, a calm demeanor, a level of assertiveness, and demonstrated coop-eration as a team player.

When you at a clinical site, be sure to make yourself known to the nursing instructor from whom you will soon need a reference letter. If you are having difficulty with a particular clinical experience, it is better if you address it first with the instructor. Let your instructor know that you want to perform better, and solicit suggestions as to how to improve. If the clinical instructor does not give out a midterm evaluation for the clinical rotation, request feedback on your own about half-way through the rotation. This will allow you time to improve your performance and also establish you in the instructor's mind as a person who is willing to ask for feedback and act on that feedback to perform at a higher level.

The more impressive the personal profile you convey to your instructor, the more impressive that instructor's sub-sequent letter of reference on your behalf will likely be. Employers also love letters from the nursing manager of the unit or facility where you are working as a nurse extern, patient care technician, or certified nurse's aide. This letter speaks about you as an employee and can catapult you to the top of the consideration list for employment.

USING YOUR NETWORK

As a nursing student, you will already have a network that can lead to a nursing job.

Start with your nursing professors. As previously noted, they have connections and advice that they will be willing to share if asked. Your clinical experiences introduced you to a team of nursing professionals, and perhaps that one nurse with whom you bonded in the skilled nursing facility or in the psych unit will be happy to hear from you as you explore job possibilities. Fellow graduates who have already found a spot in nursing will often be eager to offer a helping hand as they see opportunities that you qualify for. Make it a point to get the contact information of at least five seniors whose graduation precedes yours, asking them up front if you can contact them in the future when you begin your own job search. If you are fortunate enough to have a part-time job in health care during school, let each nurse and manager know that you will soon be graduating and would like to land a full-time position. Even non-nursing acquaintances can have a friend or neighbor who works in a place that you are interested in joining.

Get the message of your need for a job amplified by directing it toward as many contacts as you can. You may be surprised at the result.

ABOUT INTERVIEWING

Remember that you are courting a future employer who will have many suitors. Be as flexible as you can in meeting employer needs.

Be flexible when the interview touches on working arrangements. To work day shift only and no weekends is the dream of nurses everywhere, but it eludes most–particularly the newer staff members. Remember that patients are sick 24 hours a day, seven days a week, including all holidays. You are the new kid on the block and will be expected to work evening and night shifts as needed. Holidays like New Year's Day, Christmas, and Fourth of July are often staffed by the newbies! This is part of the process in most professions demanding round the clock coverage. The new hires are expected to "serve their dues" before themselves earning the right to the daytime weekday schedule.

Be flexible about where your first job will place you. By the time they graduate, many nursing students will have developed an affinity for a particular nursing specialty. Here is a tip for you. Don't start out an interview or application form restricting your availability only to critical care units, the operating room, the emergency department, or any other specialty area. If a known vacancy exists–great. But the truth is that relatively few new graduates go directly from nursing school to nursing specialty. Why? Many experienced nurses will tell you that it is not in your (or your patients') best interest to go directly from nursing school to these specialized areas. You need to absorb a lot of information and hone newly acquired skills in your first few years on the job. Working in areas where you will build a broad knowledge base while polishing organizational skills is arguably best done caring for people who are not critically ill. Generalizing before specializing will serve both you and your future patients very well.

In short, nurse recruiters are longing for the new grad who is flexible about working hours and units, have some prior health care experience besides their nursing school curriculum, and have anecdotal evidence of having demonstrated compassion, commitment, and maturity in their patient care.

When invited for an interview, know what lies ahead. Your initial interview may be with a panel (three to five people) whose job is to ascertain which new grads are worthy of a second interview. Recent grads who have landed a job say that the employer is looking for a poised, mature, well-spoken new nurse who will represent their facility and its mission to the public in a calm and professional manner. When possible, practice your interview technique at the career center or even with family or friends. Have them pose questions (that you can supply if needed) and role play. If you are somewhat shy or timid, turn the assertiveness dial up a notch or two (but no higher!) If your personality tends to be high on the excitement scale, turn the bubbly button down a notch or two (but no lower!).

What type of interview questions might you expect? Questions about your goals, your strengths and weaknesses, your flexibility, and knowledge of current issues affecting health care can be anticipated. Do an Internat search and read a few articles on current health care issues, and try to relate their impact to the health care facility you are seeking employment with.

Behavior-based questions are often used to assess your poise and ability to articulate. Remember that as a representative of the facility you will be expected to think and answer "on the spot" with patients and their families. For instance, you could be asked to describe a challenging experience you had with a patient during your nursing clinical experience and how you handled it. Or, you could be asked to describe a hurdle that you have overcome in the past. Some questions are rather blunt, such as asking what you think you can contribute to the facility.

The interview is your opportunity to allow the committee members to feel comfortable with you and to establish some rapport with them. In this culture, direct eye contact is important. Take an occasional deep breath and think before you speak. You are not being asked to fit the most words into a 60-second spot. Thinking and breathing before you speak often gives you the time to collect a thought or two and displays to the committee that you do think before you act. If you truly do not have an answer to a question or feel stymied at the moment, admit it in a calm, friendly manner. Say something like, "Well, I must admit that I never thought of that question in that way before, and I would need more time to think about my honest response. Can we return to that question later?"

After the interview, thank the panel. Inquire what the next steps in the process may be and the decision timetable. Get the names or business cards of at least the recruiter so you can thank the recruiter and all the members of the committee who were present. You can write their names down at the interview and search the web for their email address later, sending a personal thank-you to each member.

Your thank-you should be brief. State your name, the date you interviewed on, and what position (nurse residency) you are seeking. To jog their memory, mention one or two brief facts about yourself that you discussed and state that you would appreciate the opportunity to work for their organization. It does not hurt to mention here the foundation for all professional interviews:

- Dress professionally – ironed black or khaki slacks (no jeans).
  Skirts, conservative dress, reasonable shoes (no flip flops).
- Minimal jewelry, hair conservatively managed (not in face and not purple or multicolored).
- Tattoos need to be covered so as not to be visible.
- Be early (go the day before for a trial run and check out the parking or take public transportation).
- Carry a portfolio with a hard copy of your resume and letters of reference and other documents you would think useful. Don't assume that all members of the interview committee have a hard copy of your resume.
- A firm handshake and sincere smile will help your cause.
- Do not take any proffered tea, water, or coffee. It only creates a potential spill situation.
- Be prepared and expect behavioral-based questions.
- Have written prepared questions of your own in your portfolio to illustrate that you have researched this institution.
- Know the employer's Mission statement and speak to it.

PERSISTENT (NOT PESTY) FOLLOW-UP

One student lamented the fact that she sent out 64 applications for jobs and heard from none. The question that must be asked here is, "Did she follow up after sending those 64 different applications?" Picture yourself being a nurse recruiter these days, being bombarded with multiple resumes and applications from future new grads across the country. What will make your application different?

One piece of advice for your job search would be to follow up on all applications. You can do so about two weeks after sending your on-line application. Make sure you record and keep a running log of all the jobs that you apply for and the contact information for each. Two weeks after submitting your application, email or call the recruiter and just inquire if the application was received and how the hiring process is proceeding. If you delivered your resume to recruiters at a job fair, remember to take one of their business cards and follow up in the same manner.

After your initial follow-up conversation or email, ask the recruiter if it is permissible to make contact again in about two or three weeks to check on the status of your application. You want to demonstrate sincere interest in working for them but also not be put in the "pest" category. There is no hard rule as to when you officially become a pest, so pay attention to the cues you get in the conversations that you do have with the recruiter.

At the same time, don't confuse being a pest with being persistent. One recent grad who did obtain a position in a large teaching hospital's intensive care unit (she had an externship in ICU) stated that she would apply biweekly to this specific hospital and did not hear anything at all for about two months. Then, one day, she received a telephone call from the recruiter who said to her, "I figured that you are really interested in working for us since I have received so many applications from you." This diligent nursing grad was able to advertise her eagerness to work without unduly impinging on the recruiter's time.

══════════════════════════════════*FAST FACTS in a NUTSHELL*

- Get to know your clinical instructors, as their letters of reference are considered important by employers.
- Inform nursing and non-nursing contacts alike of your desire to find a nursing position. Casting a wide net will increase your job possibilities.
- Professional interview protocol is expected by prospective employers. Prepare for your interview, project professionalism and poise, and follow up with a thank-you and periodic requests for an update regarding the hiring decision.

17

Reaching for the Next Star

INTRODUCTION

In your efforts to find a job following graduation, do not lose sight of another opportunity that your nursing education has qualified you for . . . more education.

In this chapter, you will learn:

1. To look ahead as a diploma nurse.
2. To look ahead as an associate degree nurse.
3. To look ahead as a baccalaureate degree nurse.
4. About certifications and continuing education programs.

As a nurse, education will be a life-long process. At a minimum, you will need further education in the form of in-house staff development programs to ensure that your skills continue to be up to date. Most state boards of nursing require approximately 30 continuing education credits every two years for license renewal. Beyond that, the door remains open to pursue additional formal education in the hope that it will increase your professional value and perhaps prepare you for greater responsibilities.

LOOKING AHEAD AS A DIPLOMA NURSE

The diploma nursing program has been in place for many years. Courses are mostly, if not exclusively, nursing related and are designed to qualify the student to sit for the state NCLEX–RN® exam. In the United States, most diploma programs are hospital based, although there are a few that operate in a community college setting. Diploma nursing programs usually require that you have completed prerequisite college level courses with an average GPA of 2.5 before you will be admitted. Diploma schools tout the more extensive clinical experience their students receive compared to what most associate and baccalaureate programs offer. A number of nursing diploma programs have closed in recent years, as evolving hiring practices have caused some difficulty for diploma grads in procuring their first nursing job. Therefore, it is advisable for diploma nurses to enroll in an *RN-to-BSN program* upon graduation.

The RN-to-BSN Program

As the name suggests, this is a program designed for the individual who is already a registered nurse but lacking the four-year college nursing degree. There are a multitude of RN-to-BSN programs now offered by colleges. Many, if not most, can be completed in approximately one or two academic years on a part-time basis. Shop around and compare what they have to offer. For example, one school offers three credit courses in five evenings with five hours each of the five evenings. While that will appeal to those who wish to move quickly along through a program, others may prefer another school's offering at a less hectic pace. Many colleges have satellite campuses in addition to the main campus, which means that there may be an RN-to-BSN program near where you live.

(continued)

The RN-to-BSN Program (*continued*)

The programs have improved tremendously compared to their early days when the RN student was required to repeat clinical courses with the regular generic students. These current programs are available online, as blended courses combining online and classroom and, of course, all classroom. Online coursework may be considered the most convenient in terms of schedule, but many RNs enjoy the actual classroom and the opportunity it offers to personally interact with instructors and fellow nurses. Schools have adapted their classroom requirements for this unique population of student. A word of caution is to be noted here. Make sure that you enroll in an RN-to-BSN program and not an RN-to-BS program. More and more employers are requiring nurses to have a college degree specifically in nursing science (BSN). An associate degree nurse continuing on to a four-year college in a major other than nursing may have significant difficulty getting hired as a nurse. In addition, if you chose to continue with your education and enroll in a master's of science program down the line, you must have an BSN to enroll in most MSN programs.

LOOKING AHEAD AS AN ASSOCIATE DEGREE NURSE

An associate degree nurse is one who has graduated from a two-year community college. The two-year program involves both classroom instruction and onsite clinical experience along with elective courses that fall outside of the realm of nursing. Community colleges offer great value in that their tuition is generally significantly less than that of four-year colleges. Moreover, the associate nursing degree qualifies you to sit for the NCLEX–RN licensing exam. As noted, however, many hospitals and other health care facilities are demanding a BSN of their prospective nurses, which may make an RN-to-BSN program a logical next step. The RN-to-BSN program is described in the preceding section.

LOOKING AHEAD AS A BACCALAUREATE DEGREE NURSE

A baccalaureate degree nurse is one who has successfully completed a four-year college program. This BSN degree qualifies the graduate to sit for the NCLEX–RN licensing exam. Obtaining your first nursing job is an easier task with a BSN degree. One reason for this is that many hospitals covet "Magnet" status (a designation of distinction), which usually requires that there be a certain percentage of BSN nurses on staff. Similarly, it will be easier to get consideration for a position in a community nursing setting with a BSN.

Some new BSN grads may consider immediately enrolling in master's level programs upon graduation. Master's of nursing science (MSN) programs currently include specialties such as nurse practitioner, clinical nurse specialist, and nurse midwife, among others (note, however, that the profession is now moving toward the doctorate in nursing practice as the entry point for advance nursing practice roles). So, is it a good idea for the BSN to continue seamlessly into an MSN program and keep the educational momentum going?

Some would say yes, but don't feel compelled to take this plunge right away (if you even take it at all). You have worked very hard to become a registered nurse. Take time for yourself, enjoy your first years as a new nurse, have fun, take vacations, and get back to your normal life with friends before continuing on to another rigorous school experience that is often accompanied by further debt. Remember that many employers will pay for continued education once you are on staff for more than a specified period. For many, that will be the most important reason to wait before moving on to graduate studies.

Why not take some time early on to ensure that you do indeed like the nursing profession? Once you are comfortable in that regard, change units a few times or go from inpatient nursing to outpatient nursing. Then you will be more equipped to choose your advanced nursing degree program wisely. Who knows? You may decide to go to law school instead of continuing in the advanced nursing degree track. Or, you may find that your initial inclination to specialize in nursing gives way to an unexpected level of satisfaction that comes to you as a staff nurse. If you find a place of employment that values its nurses and works as a team in meeting the needs of its patients, the personal rewards of the bedside nurse will continue to pay dividends throughout your career.

And if you do proceed in your pursuit of nursing specialization, be sure to see what is required in terms of prerequisite nursing experience. You may learn that moving immediately into a nursing specialty following graduation is not always an option. For example, the new nurse who aspires to be a nurse anesthetist will find that most programs will not even consider an applicant without a minimum of two years of critical care nursing experience. And most critical care areas will not take on a nurse without at least a few years of medical-surgical experience.

CERTIFICATIONS AND CONTINUING EDUCATION PROGRAMS

There are several paths to obtain certification in a specialty area as a registered nurse. Many do not require additional formal education but do require specific continuing education in your specialized field.

American Nurses Credentialing Center

The American Nurses Credentialing Center (ANCC) is the largest credentialing center for nurses in the United States (www.nursecredentialing.org) and they offer certifications for registered nurses and advance practice nurses. Some examples of the certifications that are available for registered nurses are ambulatory care nursing, cardiac rehab nurse, cardiac vascular nursing, community health nursing, general nursing practice, home health, med-surg nursing, pediatric, pain management, etc. These types of certifications often make you eligible to move up the clinical ladder and receive more financial remuneration at your place of employment.

American Association of Critical Care Nurses

The American Association of Critical Care Nurses (AACN) offers its own credentialing program specifically for critical care nurses. Like the ANA/ANCC, an AACN credential requires a qualifying examination and has its own set of requirements that RNs must meet in order to take the credentialing examination. Critical care nurses without baccalaureate degrees in nursing are also eligible to earn certification for adult, neonatal, and pediatric critical care nurses (CCRNs). The AACN also offers a clinical specialist credential (CCNS) for master's prepared RNs and national acute care nurse practitioners (ACNPs). AACN credentials are valid for three years and are renewable. For more details on AACN credentialing, visit either the AACN or AACN's Certification Corporation.

Other Professional Nursing Associations in Specialty Practice Areas

A host of professional nursing associations representing specialty areas have their own credentialing programs. Some compete with the credentials offered by the ANA/ANCC. Others provide credentials for nurses in specialties for which the ANA/ANCC does not have an equivalent.

A few examples of certification programs offered by specialty organizations are as follow:

Nursing Specialty	Certification Program Authority
Diabetes educators	National Certification Board for Diabetes Educators
Emergency nursing	Board of Certification for Emergency Nursing
Gastroenterology nursing	American Board of Certification for Gastroenterology Nurses
HIV/AIDS nursing	HIV/AIDS Nursing Certification Board
Infectious disease nursing	Certification Board of Infection Control and Epidemiology
Infusion nursing	Infusion Nurses Certification Corporation
OB/GYN, maternal, neonatal nursing	National Certification Corporation
Oncology nursing	Oncology Nursing Certification Corporation
Pain management	American Academy of Pain Management
Perioperative nursing	Competency and Credentialing Institute
Plastic surgical nursing	American Society of Plastic Surgical Nursing
Peri- and post-anesthesia nursing	American Board of Perianesthesia Nursing Certification
School nursing	National Board of Certification for School Nurses

CONTINUING EDUCATION PROGRAMS

Most state boards of nursing require a minimum number of continuing education units to maintain licensure. This means that you will need to complete approximately 30 contact hour credits over a two-year period before you renew your nursing license. The type of programs that you can complete can be in person for a day of continuing education, online programs, or completing a nursing journal program. In terms of the latter, you can obtain continuing education credits upon completion of the questionnaire that follows at the end of the article by submitting it online or to the designated mailing address along with the required payment.

There are many sources of continuing education for nurses. Pay attention to what your state's board of nursing requires for license renewal. For instance, the board in your state may want a certain number of pharmacology or ethics credits. You can go to your state's license renewal Web site to find the specific material and credits needed for nursing. In addition to keeping your knowledge base up to date, these continuing education programs are opportunities to socialize (when you go with friends) and network (as you interact with other workshop participants).

Keep track of all programs completed, and add pertinent continuing education credits to your resume. For example, if your goal is to ultimately work in a critical care unit, take continuing education courses pertinent to critical care such as electrocardiogram or lab value interpretation, end-of-life issues, and ethics as they involve treatment of the intensive care patient. When the time comes to apply for a critical care nursing job, you will stand out as an applicant who is interested in critical care by virtue of having taken the initiative to prepare for that transition.

Finally, most nurses will be required to maintain a certification in life support throughout their careers that is received through the following programs:

American Heart Association (AHA)

All nurses are required by their employers to maintain their basic cardiopulmonary resuscitation (CPR) certification. The specific type needed is health care provider.

Advanced Cardiovascular Life Support Course (ACLS)

The extended ACLS course is designed for intensive care unit, cardiac care unit, and emergency department nurses and other health care providers who either direct or participate in the resuscitation of a patient, whether in or out of hospital. The ACLS course requires approximately 13½ hours and allows providers to enhance their skills in the treatment of the adult victim of a cardiac arrest or other cardiopulmonary emergencies using simulated clinical scenarios.

Pediatric Advanced Life Support Course (PALS)

The 14-hour PALS course provides pediatric nurses and other health care providers with information needed to recognize, prevent, and resuscitate/stabilize infants and children at risk for or experiencing cardiopulmonary arrest.

═══════════════════════════*FAST FACTS in a NUTSHELL*

- Pursuit of additional education and knowledge will be ongoing throughout your nursing career.
- Having a bachelor's degree in nursing is beneficial in pursuing job opportunities.
- Certification and continuing education programs will enhance your confidence and marketability.

18

What? Me Publish?

INTRODUCTION

Of all of the ways to distinguish yourself as a nurse, publishing is one of the most effective and least utilized. Although a resume full of degrees, certifications, and awards can open doors to getting your thoughts into print, the fact is that any current or aspiring member of the nursing profession can be an author.

In this chapter, you will learn:

1. About nursing and the publishing world.
2. About mining your personal archives.
3. About getting your name out there.

As individuals, each of us has a unique perspective. As nurses, each of us has the opportunity to share that unique perspective with others in the nursing profession via the printed word. Whether it is a highly specialized topic supported by quantitative analysis or simply an opinion based on nothing more than a meaningful patient encounter, there is potential interest among your peers in what you have to say.

ABOUT NURSING AND THE PUBLISHING WORLD

Arguably, there may be no other profession that offers one so many opportunities to publish. Take a look on the Internet and note the wide variety of journals, magazines, and newsletters that beckon to nurses.

Scholarly journals that are published by the nursing honor society Sigma Theta Tau and other nursing organizations have stringent publishing criteria and are most interested in research. Some appeal to nurses in a specialty field such as *Critical Care Nurse*. Others contain valuable updated informational articles on topics like "The Latest Developments in Diabetes Care." Reading one or even a few of these nursing publications on a regular basis is a wonderful way, if not the best way, to keep apprised of the latest trends being experienced and impacts being felt in the nursing profession. What is the latest development in research for the treatment of breast cancer? How can you recognize depression in a patient? What will recent legislation mean to the reimbursement of nurse practitioners? By keeping yourself well informed, you quietly begin to groom yourself for professional advancement.

Be forewarned that if you aspire to be published in a scholarly or peer-reviewed journal, the process is labor intensive and may not be a realistic goal for an undergraduate nursing student with a heavy school workload. Also know that these sources often expect a high level of credentials from their authors. Given that constraint, you may want to partner with a willing professor whose profile is sufficient to gain the interest of the publisher. That increases your opportunity for print access while at the same time lightening the related workload for you.

Additionally, most states have one or two complimentary magazines that are delivered in the mail or made available online to registered nurses. These magazines are financially supported by the advertisements that are contained within them. While not at the scholarly level of the journals mentioned earlier, they nonetheless are good sources of topical information. Another particular value of these nursing magazines is the listing of available nursing positions in the area, as health care entities obviously prefer to spend their recruiting dollars by reaching a targeted audience. Complimentary magazines offer short articles that may include the latest in infection prevention (for nursing credit) and patient stories.

Within this latter category lies the hidden potential for you to publish. Consider using this forum to offer opinion and insight through letters to the editor or even articles emanating from your own personal perspective. One need not be an aspiring Ernest Hemingway to be a successful nurse author. You simply need a subject that will be of interest to other nurses, a logical and thoughtful presentation of your ideas and feelings, and of course the good writing mechanics you learned long before you became a nursing student. Publishing is about having an interest, having a point, and having a willingness to share it.

The editors of these more informal publications are generally receptive to submissions by nursing students. You can contact the editor of the magazine by email and send an "inquiry" note. An inquiry is a brief letter that describes who you are and what you want to have published in their magazine or journal. The editors usually respond to this contact with a message such as, "Send it in and we will see." As mentioned in Chapter 10, one nursing student was personally touched by her care of a World War II veteran during her clinical rotation. She subsequently wrote an article about it, describing in a vivid and poignant way how this once sturdy soldier who had stormed the beach at Normandy on D-Day was now so weak and reliant on those nurses caring for him. The article was well received, and actually led her to begin volunteering her time as a nurse accompanying World War II veterans to their memorial in Washington, D.C.—serving those who decades ago crossed an ocean to serve their country.

MINING YOUR PERSONAL ARCHIVES

You will be required to write a number of term papers and other shorter opinion pieces during your nursing school education. In fact, many nursing courses are considered "writing intensive courses" for this very reason. You also may be required to write journals for many of your clinical rotations. Nursing journals can range from a two-page "how did I feel about the experience" piece to a fifteen-page thorough investigation of the patient's disease, pathophysiology, medications, assessment, and a self-reflection component. Along the way, there may be a piece of your writing that you are especially proud of. Your instructor may have commented on this writing, exclaiming that it is excellent and well-written. Why not try to publish this "masterpiece" in a nursing magazine? You may need to shorten it if it is currently a bit too long for the busy nurse who will ultimately read it. Conversely, you may choose to enhance a short self-reflection from your required journal and submit it for publishing consideration. Either way, you are leveraging your work to satisfy a class assignment and then giving it much greater visibility among your nursing colleagues.

GETTING YOUR NAME OUT THERE

As a nursing student or graduate, you are contending with many demands on your time. So why think about "getting your name out there" in the publishing world?

- You have important things to say! Possibly no one thought of writing or expressing themselves about a specific nursing event as you have done.
- It could be the beginning of a future sideline for you over the course of your career as a registered nurse.
- You need to procure your first nursing job! In a challenging job market, you will stand out as a published author, which may be the ticket to get you your first job interview or your first job.
- Last, you will experience the thrill of seeing your name in print in a magazine or journal and sharing this accomplishment with your friends and family members.

So think about getting your name out there, and letting the nursing community know who you are.

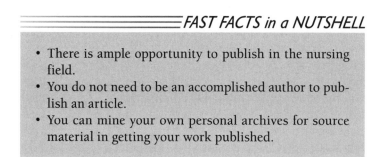

FAST FACTS in a NUTSHELL

- There is ample opportunity to publish in the nursing field.
- You do not need to be an accomplished author to publish an article.
- You can mine your own personal archives for source material in getting your work published.

19

Insuring Your Investment

INTRODUCTION

What do your health, your car, and even the dwelling you live in have in common? They should be insured. Each of these vitally important personal items is subject to loss or harm, and you need to protect yourself financially if that should occur. Remember to add your nursing license to that list.

In this chapter, you will learn:

1. About your financial exposure as a nurse.
2. About malpractice insurance.
3. About compassion as an antidote to a lawsuit.

Today's litigious society does not exclude nurses as potential defendants. Yes, they may belong to the most trusted of professions but that does not mean they are immune from lawsuits initiated by patients and patients' families. You may think that you will be covered by the institution you are employed with and that may be true. Realistically, however, you should not expect your employer alone to defend your hard-earned license and professional livelihood.

YOUR FINANCIAL EXPOSURE AS A NURSE

As you step across the threshold of your exciting new nursing career, take a moment to think about protecting your professional well-being. Investigate the need and cost of your own professional malpractice insurance (also known as liability insurance). Your employer usually will provide its nurses with some level of malpractice insurance. Remember, though, that this insurance will only cover you in your actions as an employee of the facility. Isn't that enough?

Not really. Conventional wisdom says that the attorneys for the institution that employs you will have the protection of the employer's reputation and finances as their primary objective. While they may do their best to defend you as a nurse if named as a defendant in a lawsuit, you may not be their top priority.

A more common potential hazard is the instance in which your nursing expertise is sought by those you know personally. Your elderly neighbor will ask your advice regarding a medication. Your long-lost cousin will call you and inquire what the bulge on her hip may mean. Your friends will visit you and tell you that they have been feeling poorly, and solicit your opinion on what to do. Will you be responsive to these questions? If you answer with a "yes," as most nurses will, keep in mind that you can be sued in the event of an adverse outcome traceable to the assistance you gave. Even when you are "off-duty," you are still legally liable because the standard nursing license does not allow you to diagnose or prescribe.

MALPRACTICE INSURANCE

Recognizing the risks as just described, it is wise to obtain your own nursing liability coverage to protect your personal assets if you were to be sued. Fortunately, nursing liability policies tend to be relatively inexpensive. Make sure that your policy specifies that it is "occurrence based." This means that you remain covered for an incident that may have occurred years before as long as the coverage was in effect at that time, and even if that same coverage was later discontinued.

Notify your malpractice insurer immediately if you are the object of a lawsuit relating to the care or advice you rendered. They will advise you not to contact the claimant and will ask you for as much detailed information as possible about the incident. As any nurse who has experienced this process will tell you, detailed and thorough notes made at the time of the occurrence are very beneficial in defending what you did and why you did it. Detailed notes of all assessments, teachings, education, safety measures, and any unexpected occurrence are required by all health care organizations. Don't succumb to the temptation to rush through them as an unimportant administrative chore. While the likelihood that they will need to be referenced in conjunction with a legal action is very small, the potential still exists!

Even as a student nurse, you need to take the time to thoroughly write your notes (usually on a computer) and check with your nurse and instructor about any unusual circumstance concerning your patient. Not surprisingly, you will be required to carry your own malpractice insurance as a student nurse.

COMPASSION: AN ANTIDOTE
TO A LAWSUIT

As a nurse, you will work hard and conscientiously to perform your duties and responsibilities with the utmost care and professionalism. And still, you may make a mistake. Ask most nurses who have practiced in the field for a significant period of time, and they will be able to recount an error that they made in the discharging of their responsibilities. Most of the time, thankfully, there is not an untoward effect on the patient, but occasionally . . .

As they say, accidents happen. When they do, what makes the difference in a patient and the family deciding whether to contact an attorney? Often one factor that will play a significant role in the patient's and family's decision to pursue legal action is their own perception regarding the compassion exhibited by the nursing staff.

"Incidents don't sue—patients do" (Stabler-Haas & McHugh, 1989). This statement is a manifestation of the fact that patients are people first. As such, nurses who incorporate compassion into the care they render can sometimes escape the snare of a malpractice suit that pulls in other staff members. Simple practices such as answering call lights quickly and apologizing when you don't, maintaining direct and open communication with the patient and his family, explaining all procedures in understandable terms, holding the patient's hand when it needs to be held, and exhibiting genuine caring in all of your interactions will heighten the personal regard that the patient and family have for you. When you realize that the emotions that lead to the family and patient filing a lawsuit center around anger and a feeling of being disregarded, it is easy to see the value of rendering compassionate nursing care. This is illustrated next.

One Result of Compassionate Care

Abby has twenty years of bedside experience as a nurse. She has worked at this hospital for the last fifteen years of her career. She is known as the nurse who will stay a few minutes after her shift and speak to a patient's family—even bringing them a cup of coffee or tea when they need a little boost. She always introduces herself when she initially enters a patient's room and explains her plans for the care she will provide. She will sit beside the patients if they are upset and just hold their hand for a few minutes to assuage any anxiety they may be feeling. She remembers to close the curtain or door when her care requires any personal exposure of patients to ensure privacy and dignity. She is known for her back rubs for patients who, despite the "wonders" of modern medicine, still are in pain. She is, quite simply, a nurse's nurse.

Unfortunately, on night shift one of her patients fell and broke her hip, requiring surgery and prolonging the hospitalization and rehabilitation. The patient's family was upset about this fall that their beloved mother had experienced and were discussing among themselves the possibility of contacting an attorney about the incident. Overhearing her family, the patient adamantly forbade her children to even consider such an act. "Abby was the nurse on duty that night. She is the best and most compassionate nurse of all and I do not want her to have any trouble about this. It was my own fault. I should have not gotten up by myself. Abby told me not to get out of bed myself and I did not listen to her. It is not her fault."

One Result of Not-So-Compassionate Care

Zena has ten years of experience as a bedside nurse. She has been employed at the hospital for the past two years. She is known to clock out of work a few minutes before the end of her shift. She rarely will talk with families of patients and has been heard in the nurses' station stating that families should be banned from visiting in the hospital. She often does not introduce herself to her patients, running into their rooms to administer medications and barely speaking as she performs her responsibilities. She talks about the patients in the hallways and elevators and at lunch in the cafeteria. She has not given a patient a back rub since her nursing school days and likes the night shift because she "does not want to deal with the families." She is brusque on the telephone when patients' family members call for an update.

(continued)

One Result of Not-So-Compassionate Care (*continued*)

Last week, her patient fell out of bed en route to the bathroom and broke his hip, which required surgery and prolonged hospitalization. The patient's family discussed the possibility of contacting an attorney upon their father's discharge. When their father heard the discussion he stated, "Yes, we should get a lawyer. That miserable nurse was on duty that night and the reason that I did not ask for assistance is that she is so unpleasant to deal with."

So an occasional back rub means that you won't be sued? You won't need liability insurance? Not at all. The point is simply that a kind word, a held hand, a few extra minutes to ensure a thorough explanation to a patient and family can make a difference and possibly protect you from a lawsuit. After all, if you were the patient who fell, how might you have reacted in each case?

============*FAST FACTS in a NUTSHELL*

- Despite the esteem in which they are held, nurses can be sued.
- Obtaining nursing liability coverage is a relatively inexpensive way to protect yourself financially.
- Compassionate nursing care can dissuade patients and their families from lawsuits.

20

A Nursing Fable

Once upon a time . . .

. . . there lived a high school student named Laura, who had graduated in the top 10% of her class. She coveted a career in health care. Perhaps she would become a chiropractor. It was after all a chiropractor who had provided her welcome relief from a back injury she suffered while playing for her school's field hockey team. So, Laura decided to declare herself a science/biology major in college. As her freshman year progressed, however, she was surprised to find that she was not getting as personally invested in her studies as she should. Laura had always enjoyed the sciences, particularly biology and chemistry, but she did not really want to take all of the science content that was required for her chosen major. Meanwhile, she began to hear compelling stories about, of all things, nursing.

Laura went to her biology adviser inquiring about the possibility of transferring in her sophomore year to nursing as her major. Her adviser, a wizened tenured professor, initially warned her that she may not be able to transfer into nursing since it is quite a competitive process. Laura, undeterred, completed the required transfer of major paperwork and made an appointment with the director of the nursing department. Laura was impressed by the nursing director, who reiterated the fact that there are a large number of potential transfer students waiting for an available spot in the university's nursing program.

To promote her own cause, Laura presented herself as a mature, responsible college student and gave the director a sample of one of her term papers that she had recently completed. Her topic was the "Disarray of the Health Care System," and she received an A grade for her work. She followed up on the discussion with a thank-you email to the director. In her message, Laura briefly summarized her personal profile and her strong desire to become a registered nurse, underscoring her interest by noting that she had been a volunteer during high school at a neighborhood hospital.

To Laura's surprise and delight she received notification in late August that she was accepted as a sophomore student into the nursing program. Since she was a biology major, she had all of the prerequisite sciences required for nursing sophomores and easily transitioned into the sophomore class, keeping on track for a four-year graduation. Her first step on becoming a nursing student was to join the student nurse association to facilitate her meeting other students in her major.

In her first student nurse association meeting, Laura learned that nursing classes were very different from biology and other classes she had taken as a freshman. The nursing professors expected the students to read before class and after class. If they did not, the student nurses quickly became lost in the fast-paced content of the classroom. There also was little time for discussion in the class since it occurred in a huge lecture hall. Several students recommended taping all lectures and then going back over the tapes after class and converting them into printed outlines and study notes. These students said that they also made an appointment with the appropriate nursing professor before each major exam, asking pertinent questions about the lecture content that would be the focus of the test. One especially friendly student invited Laura to join his study group.

To sustain her concentration during lectures, Laura began to bring a lunch bag to her nursing classes, which lasted for four hours straight. She brought a sandwich, banana, and a diet soda, which allowed her to remain focused for the four-hour lecture period. Laura was successful in her first nursing exam but then became quickly concerned during her next nursing module—the renal system and disease, feeling that she was completely lost and did not understand what the nursing professor was trying to teach. In her new study group she realized that her peers had a much better understanding of the renal content. She quickly made an appointment with the instructor and brought a list of specific questions with her so the instructor would observe that she had worked hard on her own to understand this content.

In the spring of her sophomore year, she entered her first clinical rotation, which occurred in a neighborhood skilled nursing facility. She did complete physical and mental health assessments and complete bed baths on several dependent elders. Laura loved the experience. In one of her nursing journals she wrote the following: "I feel as though I forget why I want to be a nurse until I am on the floor and with a patient." She experienced the personal satisfaction that only occurs in clinical rotations. Touching a stranger and offering healing was truly what inspired Laura to transfer and pursue nursing. While she learned the science of nursing and biology in the classroom, the art of nursing can only be learned in a real clinical site.

Her experience at the clinical site caring for real patients taught Laura an unexpected lesson. She learned that patients' mental health can have as much to do with their physical health as any other factor. This observation led her to begin inquiring about her clients' level of sadness and level of interest in their usual activities. Laura discovered that many people lying in hospital beds with abdominal pain of unknown cause had an undercurrent depression or anxiety. She continued to note these connections and planned to continue to assess her clients' physical and mental health status and their interconnections. She began to read about mindfulness-based stress reduction as an antidote for chronic pain and an adjunct to living a more full and present life.

Laura became fast friends with the staff at the skilled nursing home and obtained a part-time job there to continue her learning and to earn extra money during the remainder of her nursing program. She also discovered much later that this experience as a nurse's aide in the skilled nursing facility became the ticket that enticed several hospitals to offer her an interview for a graduate nurse position upon graduation.

One of her friends had a very different experience than Laura during his first clinical experience. Joe had a medical-surgical clinical experience at a local hospital. On his first day, a patient care technician (PCT) "yelled" at him for approaching so abruptly and not introducing himself. Joe felt like he was being singled out and that he only asked a question for the welfare of his patient. Laura and Joe met after clinical to discuss Joe's experience. Joe admitted to Laura that he did not introduce himself to the PCT, but rather just plunged into his conversation requesting that she do the "AccuChek" immediately so he could administer insulin to his patient. Laura reminded Joe that students are guests at each clinical site, and that as a guest he must introduce himself and make sure that it is a convenient time to make his inquiry. Another student joined in the discussion, saying that she felt that she made a mistake pursuing nursing since her first patient directed her to "leave the room" when she entered. Laura inquired more about the situation and learned that this student did not ask about the patient's pain level, and immediately began to pull the patient's legs and arms to assess his range of motion. Upon further inquiry, they all discovered that this patient had severe rheumatoid arthritis and that, in the morning, his pain is at its worst. It would be better to visit the patient, give him something for pain, and come back in half an hour to complete an assessment.

One of Laura's closest friends failed in her sophomore year in the nursing program and would be required to repeat the spring semester of her sophomore year. Laura was concerned and met her friend for lunch one day to talk about it. Her friend told Laura that she was working 30 hours a week at a nearby restaurant while being full-time in the nursing program, often not getting to bed until 2:00 a.m. before clinical days. While her friend needed the money, she now realized it is more expensive to repeat a whole semester in school. The friend now lamented the fact that she had worked so much. Laura thought to herself how she was glad that she heeded her mother's words to get enough sleep, food, and some fun during this rigorous course of study. Laura suggested that her friend visit the counseling center and walked her over to it. Her friend was feeling very depressed about the need to repeat her sophomore semester and vaguely hinting that life was not worth continuing at this point. Laura was astute enough to know that comments like these could not go unaddressed.

Laura spent one hour a week as a sophomore student in her nursing program's computer lab reviewing NCLEX® questions that the director of the lab had set up for them. Many of her classmates poked fun at her for doing this so early in the program, but Laura had read that the sooner one gets accustomed to NCLEX questions and practicing in an environment other than their own bedroom, the greater is the prospect of success in passing on the first try. She also went to the career counseling office in her junior year to create a resume and received other vital tips on obtaining a job on graduation.

Laura's regimen was resulting in good grades up through senior year, at which time she began her job search. Although she had not yet graduated, Laura applied to five facilities—four acute care hospitals and one skilled nursing home. She stated in her application that she would be happy to work on any floor or any shift, including weekends as a new employee. She emphasized how she enjoyed the philosophy of each institution that she applied to (after looking up their mission statement online), including a piece of it in her letter of application. Laura had wisely requested letters of recommendation from her clinical instructors immediately after each clinical rotation for eventual use in her job search. She knew that these same instructors would be bombarded in the late fall of her senior year when the rest of her classmates realized how vital these letters become in the pursuit of a nursing graduate position. She was offered interviews at three of her choices and purchased a new navy blue suit for the interviews. She dressed conservatively, developed thoughtful questions to pose at each interview, and took care to ensure that she was not feeling hungry or fatigued when she met with each prospective employer.

The interviewers asked her different behavioral situation questions. "Tell us what you will offer to our institution?" "What evidence-based practice topic would you like to initiate as a nurse in our facility?" "What has been your most rewarding patient encounter during your student experience?" Fortunately, Laura had the foresight to have practiced responding to such questions with her roommate. As a result, she was well prepared and presented herself as a poised, articulate young woman.

Laura was offered two different positions in April of her senior year. She chose to accept the medical-surgical nursing position at a nearby teaching hospital. While she was not sure what path she would pursue later as a nurse, she knew that the skills of organization and acquiring knowledge about a myriad of different disease processes along with their care would position her well to pursue almost any path later in her nursing career. For a graduation gift, Laura asked her parents to purchase her own individual malpractice insurance to protect her educational investment and also to pay for the NCLEX review course. As a result of her careful planning and hard work, she passed the boards on her first attempt and took a week off down at the beach before beginning her hospital orientation program.

And Laura worked as a registered nurse happily ever after.

In Student Nurses' Own Words . . .

"I took any part-time job that I could, working doing physicals, or filling in for other nurses until I landed this job. All those other part-time experiences helped me get this job and I wouldn't have thought it possible when I first graduated. I love it."

"Every clinical experience that you encounter throughout your program can and may be treated like a job interview. By showing enthusiasm and commitment to nursing as a profession, you are making connections, practicing your interviewing skills, and learning as much as possible."

"In applying for my license, I did everything online. The one big thing I had trouble with was that I showed up at the NCLEX test site with the wrong paperwork and I was not able to take the test on the day I had scheduled! I had printed out the wrong thing as a test voucher."

"I was hired with three other new grads. Every one of us had been aides on the unit."

"Don't 'settle' for a job. I know a few other people who took jobs wherever they could and now they're stuck in a specialty that they don't enjoy."

"I largely attribute my RN position to the connections I made during my externship after junior year."

"Some people loved the classroom review for NCLEX, but me not so much. I passed the boards using a flash card review system with over 1200 questions arranged by clinical area and body system. Each card had the answer along with complete rationale. I could basically study anywhere."

"If you are able to get an externship, stay in touch with management and recruiters of that site throughout the year. Be persistent, but not annoying."

"Nurses need to have a regular self-care routine (nutrition, adequate sleep, stress-relieving methods, exercise) in order to avoid burnout."

"The night before the NCLEX I did not study. I treated myself to a pedicure, Chinese food, and sleep. I passed on the first attempt."

"I did get a temporary practice permit, but my job did not accept that to work as an RN so basically it was a waste of money for me."

"Calling and talking to someone at the state nursing board was a big help in getting my questions about the licensing process answered."

References

Della Cava, M. (2011, March 11). *USA Today.*

Goleman, D. (2006). *Emotional intelligence: 10th anniversary edition: Why it can matter more than I.Q.* New York: Bantam Dell.

Nafziger, B. (2010). *Nurses most trusted profession for the 11th year: Gallup Poll.* Retrieved March 5, 2011, from dotmed.com/news/story/14916

National Council for State Boards of Nursing. (2011). Retrieved August 4, 2011, from https://www.ncsbn.org/index.htm

National League for Nursing. (2011). *Annual survey of schools of nursing.* Retrieved August 10, 2011, from nln.org/research/slides/pdf/as0809

Reilly, D., & Oermann, M. (1992). *Clinical teaching in nursing education.* New York: National League for Nursing.

Robert Wood Johnson Foundation. (2011). *Enrollment growth continues at baccalaureate and graduate level nursing schools.* Retrieved April 25, 2011, from rwjf.org/healthpolicy/quality/product

Stabler-Haas, S., & McHugh, M. (1989). Compassion: A strategy for avoiding a lawsuit. *Critical Care Nurse, 9*(2), 12–14.

Stokowski, L. (2011, June 17). *Looking out for our new nurse grads: What happened to the jobs?* Retrieved September 29, 2011, from http://www.medscape.com

Index

AACN. *See* American Association of Critical Care Nurses
Academic support course, 126
ACLS. *See* Advanced Cardiovascular Life Support Course
ACNPs. *See* Acute care nurse practitioners
Acute care nurse practitioners (ACNPs), 154
Advance for Nurses, 85
Advanced Cardiovascular Life Support Course (ACLS), 157
AHA. *See* American Heart Association
American Association of Critical Care Nurses (AACN), 154
American Heart Association (AHA), 156
American Nurses Credentialing Center (ANCC), 153–154
American Psychological Association (APA), 34
Anatomy and physiology course, 18

ANCC. *See* American Nurses Credentialing Center
APA. *See* American Psychological Association
Assistants, nursing, 77
Associate degree nurse, 151
"Authorization to Test" letter, 120

Baccalaureate degree nurse, 152–153
Barton, Clara, 52
Behavior-based questions, 145
Biology course, 18
Breathing exercise, 111

Cardiopulmonary resuscitation (CPR) certification, 67, 156
Career development center, services offered by, 135
CCNS. *See* Clinical specialist credential
CCRNs. *See* Critical care nurses
CDC. *See* Centers for Disease Control and Prevention

186   INDEX